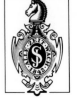

Rolf Inderbitzi

Surgical Thoracoscopy

With Forewords by U. Althaus
and C. Boutin

With 50 Figures, mostly in Colour,
in 92 Parts

Springer-Verlag

Berlin Heidelberg New York
London Paris Tokyo
Hong Kong Barcelona
Budapest

Dr. Rolf Inderbitzi
Head of the surgical department
Spital Limmattal

8952 Schlieren-Zürich
Switzerland

Title of the German Edition:
Chirurgische Thorakoskopie
© Springer-Verlag Berlin Heidelberg 1993

ISBN 3-540-56894-8
Springer-Verlag Berlin Heidelberg New York

ISBN 0-387-56894-8
Springer-Verlag New York Berlin Heidelberg

Library of Congress Cataloging-in-Publication Data. Inderbitzi, Rolf, 1954– [Chirugische thorakoskopie. English] Surgical thoracoscopy / Rolf Inderbitzi ; with forewords by U. Althaus and C. Boutin. p. cm. Includes bibliographical references and index. ISBN 3-540-56894-8 (alk. paper).— ISBN 0-387-56894-8 (alk. paper) 1. Chest—Endoscopic surgery. 2. Thoracoscopy. I. Title. [DNLM: 1. Pleural Diseases—diagnosis. 2. Pleural Diseases—surgery. 3. Thoracic Surgery—methods. 4. Thoracoscopy—methods. WF 700 I38c 1993a] RD536.I5313 1993 617.5'4059—dc20

© Springer-Verlag Berlin Heidelberg 1994
Printed in Germany

Typesetting: Best-set Typesetter Ltd., Hong Kong
24/3130 – 5 4 3 2 1 0 – Printed on acid-free paper

For Christine, Andreas and Laura

Foreword – Surgery

In recent decades, surgical practice saw the development of operating techniques which subjected patients to large incisions and allowed the surgeon fast, unhindered and comfortable access to the target organ. Endoscopic surgery was slow to gain a footing and, being denigrated as unworthy "keyhole surgery", it was not taken seriously in surgical circles. Even for diagnostic purposes, endoscopy was seldom used in the thoracic cavity.

R. Inderbitzi was one of the first European surgeons to recognize the surgical potential of endoscopy in thoracic surgery. Despite sceptical comments from colleagues, he did not waver in his conviction that the chest was a preformed body cavity that was suitable for therapeutic thoracoscopic measures. In numerous, systematic investigations in the Department of Pathology at the University of Bern, he developed a series of new instruments adapted to the particular anatomical situation in the thorax. With this instrument set it was possible to extend the previous range of indications for interventional thoracoscopy considerably. Dr. Inderbitzi's greatest contribution was, however, the introduction of video techniques into thoracoscopic surgery. Impressed by the success of minimally invasive surgery in the abdominal cavity and recognizing the advantages of electronic image transmission, a technique that was already well-established in this area, he paved the way for the spatial separation of image and operating field in thoracoscopy. The new-found ability to record the image electronically and to transmit it to a monitor is one of the main reasons behind the new impulses we have recently witnessed in thoracoscopy.

This monograph provides a comprehensive review of the current situation in thoracoscopic surgery, which has been greatly influenced by R. Inderbitzi. The various techniques determined by the indications and the results achieved by the author are clearly described and interpreted in numerous tables and illustrations. The book reflects considerable dedication and is an informative source of reference for pneumologists and thoracic surgeons alike.

U. Althaus
Bern, November 1992

Foreword – Pneumology

Thoracoscopy is in a phase of rapid evolution: 1992 was proclaimed as thoracoscopy year by the American Pneumology Congress. Hardly a week goes by without specialists coming together somewhere at congresses and seminars. New indications follow one after the other in quick succession, ranging from interventions on the pleura and lung and extending to the pericardium and mediastinum. Developments in endoscopic technology are the prime reason for such progress, allowing interventions that would not have been possible even in the recent past.

Thoracoscopy was developed in 1910 by the Swedish internist Jacobaeus, who described both thoracoscopy and laparoscopy. His endoscope was a cystoscope which had been developed shortly before by Georg Wolf (father of Richard Wolf). His intention was to divide adhesive bands in order to improve the usual form of contemporary treatment of tuberculosis by inducing a complete pneumothorax. Even in those early days, he used thermocautery and a telescope with a straight and lateral field of view. The intervention was performed without anaesthesia or antibiotics.

Interventions of this type were performed up until the 1950s on both sides of the Atlantic. In Europe it was the pneumologists and in the USA the surgeons who performed such thoracoscopies known as pneumolysis or Jacobaeus' operation.

With the introduction of tuberculostatic agents, the technique was largely lost and practically ceased to be taught. Nevertheless, a few remained true to thoracoscopy: Brandt and later Loddenkemper in Berlin, Swieringa and later Vanderschueren in Utrecht and Sattler in Vienna were pioneers of this technique to which Jacobaeus had already ascribed a large number of diagnostic and therapeutic advantages. All were still using endoscopes illuminated by a simple light bulb.

Since then, thoracoscopic technology has developed in leaps and bounds. The cold light source became available in the second half of the 1960s, and we have now also been involved in improving the instruments ourselves. From that time onwards, instrument development gained ever-increasing impetus. Space research promoted innovation in electronics such as video technology, which in turn stimulated the imagination of researchers who found industry willing and able to implement their ideas.

In this respect, Dr. R. Inderbitzi played an important and original role. He was the first to realize that angled instruments would allow optimum dissection in a concave cavity. As simple as the idea may be, it had to be first thought of and then proved. Time has shown that he was right, and the use of forceps, scissors and hooks such as these through special trocar sleeves makes all the corners and recesses of the pleural cavity accessible.

Dr. Inderbitzi's experience is remarkable. We had the opportunity to admire his ability when he took part in a symposium we organized in Marseilles in October 1991. He has performed a large number of wide-ranging thoracoscopic interventions and can certainly be counted among the world's leading thoracoscopic surgeons. He was also one of the first to realize that the introduction of minimally invasive techniques would bring about fundamental changes in thoracic surgery.

Pneumology should also be receptive to these stimulating ideas and follow a similar course. Diagnostic and therapeutic interventions such as placing pleural drainage tubes, diagnostic thoracoscopy for pleurisy and diffuse pulmonary disease and therapeutic thoracoscopy for relapsing pleural effusions and spontaneous pneumothorax are familiar to the pneumologist. With thorough technical knowledge, the techniques used are safe – even in the hands of internists, in contrast to the opinions of some American surgeons. I have personally performed more than 2500 thoracoscopies and never required assistance of a surgeon.

The situation in Europe and the USA, however, hardly bears comparison. Would it not be more worthwhile to promote and develop co-operation between internists and surgeons instead of observing strict lines of demarcation and stressing the different positions? There is no good reason why well-trained pneumologists should do without modern and efficient equipment and continue to use outdated instruments and units. In our opinion, there is nothing to prevent co-operation between internists and surgeons while still maintaining the traditional indications. Surgeons have always been more interested in the treatment of tumours than in pleural disease. Internists should continue to use thoracoscopy for diagnostic purposes and for performing pleurodesis. The same can be said for spontaneous pneumothorax, which is often not a surgical indication. These patients can generally also be treated thoracoscopically and without difficulty by pneumologists. Abrasion of the pleura and talc pleurodesis are efficient and not difficult to perform. If, on the other hand, resection of bullae or a parietal pleurectomy is necessary, this is clearly a surgical intervention. With adequate experience and skill, the pneumologist is also capable of performing other thoracoscopic interventions. Dorsal sympathectomy, for example, and pericardial and pulmonary biopsy can be categorized as technically simple manoeuvres which can be performed quickly.

If more complex techniques are required in occasional cases, these are then the province of the surgeon. The traditional indications for thoracic surgery must not go unmentioned. Many of these will, in future, be approached using minimally invasive techniques.

Let us hope that dedication to our task as physicians and our responsibility to our patients will ensure that dialogue and co-operation between pneumologists and surgeons will be at the forefront where we share common interests.

C. Boutin
Marseilles, November 1992

Acknowledgements

Turning an idea into reality and writing a book about the results is only possible when a whole series of circumstances are favourable and when many people are selflessly prepared to lend their help and creativity. My heartfelt thanks to all those supporters.

First and foremost, I would like to thank my former head of department, Professor U. Althaus, Director of the Department of Thoracic and Cardio-vascular Surgery of the University Hospital Bern, for his trust and generosity in allowing me the time and providing the opportunity to set up the infrastructure required to introduce surgical thoracoscopy in Bern. Professors U. Althaus, B. Nachbur and P. Stirnemann were also my mentors and advised and guided me in the most important aspects of thoracic surgery. I must also thank my medical colleagues and H. Gilgen from the Department of Pathology at the University of Bern, who not only made sure I had the peace and quiet necessary to carry out preclinical investigations and measurements, but also often provided active support. The evaluation of thoracoscopy according to the principles of minimally invasive surgery would not have been possible without the untiring support of the firm of Treier Endoskopie AG, Beromünster, Switzerland. R. Treier was always ready to lend a helping hand and give his support whenever needed. In constant consultation with H. Heckele, the experienced head of development of the firm of Richard Wolf, Knittlingen, Germany, the preconditions for clinical application of the method were satisfied without delay.

The unqualified support of the department of internal medicine of the University Hospital under the direction of Professors H. Studer and

W. Straub meant that the conversion to clinical application did not go through a slow and tedious start-up phase, but permitted over 100 thoracoscopies to be performed in the first year. Receptive to our arguments regarding possible indications, our internist colleagues referred many patients to us. From the very beginning we were in close contact with the pneumological department under Professor H. Bachofen and were thankful for much expert advice. The fast introduction of surgical thoracoscopy into the daily routine of pulmonary surgery without major complications would not have been possible without the dedication of Professor D. Thomson's anaesthetists and the co-operation of the nursing staff under Sister Barbara Stähli, who patiently tested new patient positions, provided constructive ideas at the operating table and carefully prepared the many and often changing instrument prototypes. The atmosphere among colleagues in our own department was reflected in a readiness to join in and to provide constructive criticism typified by the selfless dedication and enthusiasm of Markus Furrer and Janosch Molnar.

The time available in the busy operating schedule of a university hospital often made patient and comprehensive photography of thoracoscopic manoeuvres impossible. The artistic talent of K. Oberli more than made up for this shortcoming. The speedy publication of this book would not have been possible without the advice and help of U. Kesselbach and his team from the firm of Richard Wolf, Knittlingen, Germany. I would also like to thank the staff of Springer-Verlag for producing this beautifully laid out book so quickly.

Final words of thanks must go to colleagues further afield, whose help was essential to the introduction of thoracoscopy in Bern and to the writing of this book. Professor C. Boutin, Marseilles, lent us his full support and great experience at an early stage of the project in Spring 1990. Professor R. Loddenkemper, Berlin, spontaneously offered to lend us slides for the book (Figs. 17b, 34, 36).

The genuine interdisciplinary co-operation between surgeons, pneumologists and internists and the close contact with colleagues abroad is for me the greatest source of pleasure to have resulted from the work of the last three years – hopefully a good omen for the future.

Such a project takes up a considerable amount of time and there is no denying that it is the family who must bear the brunt. This book is dedicated to them with deeply felt gratitude.

R. Inderbitzi
Schlieren-Zürich, November 1992

Contents

B   Specific Techniques

Introduction

Minimally invasive surgery is currently experiencing a hectic period of development in terms of operating techniques, instruments and technology. Thorough, well-founded knowledge of these new techniques is nevertheless still almost completely absent. Even with techniques as widely accepted as endoscopic cholecystectomy, there are still no long-term results available to allow comparisons with the traditional "open" methods. Only after thorough studies encompassing all patients and precise documentation of the clinical results will the method be able to take its place as an established procedure in traditional surgery. This book represents a resumé of the current situation in surgical thoracoscopy and will hopefully serve to provoke new discussion.

Following thoracotomy, early postoperative pain and associated respiratory restrictions with their attendant risks are often a serious problem for the patient. Reducing the size of the site of entry is a logical surgical solution to this problem, and it is made possible by thoracoscopy. This method allows a comprehensive view of the pleural cavities via mini-incisions. High-resolution endoscopes with small diameters, video cameras and monitors which are constantly being improved, and the development of a large number of suitable instruments have made such surgical interventions possible. The semi-rigid thoracic cavity and its anatomical structures are ideally suited for minimally invasive methods. Many surgical/technical problems nevertheless remain unsolved. There is, for example, no substitute for the probing, exploring fingers of the surgeon, which represents a greater disadvantage in the minimally invasive surgery of soft tissue than it does, for example, in arthroscopic surgery, where the manual palpation of ligaments or menisci is of little importance.

In addition to relying on existing experience and techniques learned from surgical laparoscopy, thoracic surgeons practising minimally invasive procedures can also draw on the decades of experience of pneumologists versed in the techniques of thoracoscopy. Discussion and a mutual exchange of information should be encouraged. "Speaking the same language" and using generally accepted divisions and classifications such as the endoscopic evaluation of spontaneous pneumothorax according to Vanderschueren [167, 168] will help to further communication and dispel prejudice.

The first part of this book deals with the standard technique we use in thoracoscopic surgery. This has been developed on the basis of initial experimental work and more than 250 interventions and is the method we use successfully today. The second part of the book describes possible indications, techniques that have found application, and results to date.

If this book provides the basis for and provokes critical discussion and promotes further interest in thoracoscopic surgery, it will have fulfilled its purpose.

A General

1 Historical Development

Thoracoscopy was first introduced by the Scandinavian internist Jacobaeus in 1912 [89]. Since then it has had changing fortunes as a diagnostic and therapeutic method. Originally conceived as a primarily diagnostic tool [89, 90], it was used mainly for pleural adhesiolysis and the establishment of an iatrogenic pneumothorax [117] in the therapy of tuberculosis until the introduction of tuberculostatic agents. With the advent of medical tuberculosis therapy, thoracoscopy increasingly became a purely diagnostic procedure. The sudden rise in the number of publications in recent years indicates a renewed interest in this method. Improved biopsy techniques with high specificity and sensitivity are useful in pneumological diagnosis [22, 24, 34, 125]. Therapeutically, the technique is used mainly by pneumologists in the treatment of malignant pleural effusions and spontaneous pneumothorax [124, 181].

F. Cova, who published an impressive colour atlas as early as 1928 [37], must be mentioned along with more recent protagonists such as A. Sattler [148, 149, 151], H. J. Brandt [26, 27] and C. Boutin [21], as pioneers and outstanding proponents of modern pneumological thoracoscopy.

In 1982, K. Semm [154], a gynaecologist, performed the first laparoscopic appendectomy. However, only after the successful performance of an endoscopic cholecystectomy in 1987 by Mouret [121] and the development and standardization of the technique in 1989 by Dubois [44], Götz [133], Klaiber [97], Pérrisat [131] and Reddick [139] was the interest of surgeons in laparoscopic surgery finally awakened. The breakthrough, when it came, was staggering and in the meantime "minimally invasive surgery", a term coined by the English urologist Wickham [185], has become the subject of meetings, workshops, congresses and courses the world over.

By comparison, endoscopic surgery of the thoracic cavity has developed calmly. Although thoracoscopic interventions have been performed successfully on the sympathetic trunk and vagus nerve for over 30 years by R. Wittmoser [188] in Germany and R. Wepf [46] in Switzerland, there was no widespread response. The time and circumstances were simply not yet right.

With the synthesis of the wide experience of pneumologists and the principles of minimally invasive surgery, and particularly the introduction of video endoscopy, the surgical possibilities of thoracoscopy have been rapidly increased. After carrying out experimental studies in 1989, we started performing operative thoracoscopy from January 1990 onwards [88]. This replaced the previous technique of exploration of the thoracic cavity using a mediastinoscope, as described by Maassen [110], and allowed increasingly complex surgical interventions, which have so far extended to successfully performed lobectomy in animals.

2 Endoscopic Anatomy

Precise knowledge of the endoscopic anatomy of the thoracic cavity is necessary before diagnostic and therapeutic thoracoscopies are performed.

The whole chest cavity is lined by the serous parietal pleura. In the area of the hilum it forms a fold and becomes the visceral pleura to cover the lungs. The parietal pleura is attached to subserous fibrous tissue, the endothoracic fascia. The pleura can be surgically detached from this fascia in an avascular layer. In the sternal and paravertebral regions, the endothoracic fascia gradually becomes the mediastinum.

The highly sensitive innervation of the parietal pleura includes the phrenic nerve (diaphragm and mediastinum) and the intercostal nerves in the region of the thoracic wall. If a thoracoscopy is performed with the patient under local anaesthesia, the operator must remember that careless contact with the parietal pleura and mediastinum can trigger severe pain. The lung and heart are controlled by the sympathetic and parasympathetic nervous systems. Traction on the lung can cause coughing as a result of stimulation of the vagus nerve; touching the heart can cause cardiac dysrhythmias such as supraventricular extrasystoles [48, 125], sinus tachycardia [125], hypotonia [38, 70] and vasovagal reactions [172].

Right Thoracic Cavity [6, 10, 71, 158] (Fig. 1)
The right lung has three lobes divided by two oblique fissures. The main fissure (fissura interlobaris obliqua) divides the superior and middle lobes from the inferior lobe. With the lung expanded, this runs approximately along the fifth rib (Fig. 2). The transverse fissure separates the superior and middle lobes. This runs lateroventrally at approximately the height of the fourth

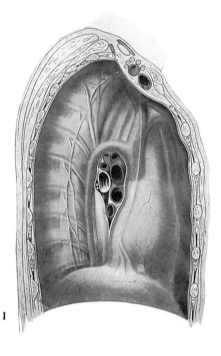

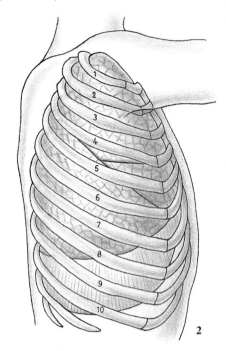

rib. The division of the lobes may be incomplete bilaterally, a situation which leads to large bridges of parenchyma forming.

    The thoracoscopic exploration begins at the height of the hilum and continues in an anti-clockwise direction. If the lung is not completely collapsed, the fissures can be used as a track to the hilum. The cone of light from the telescope glides over the pulmonary vein covered by the visceral pleura to the pericardium. Heart movements can be clearly recognized. On the pericardium the phrenic nerve can be seen as a white cord. This nerve runs from cranial to caudal on the vena cava over the pericardium to the diaphragm. At the height of the thoracic inlet, the vagus nerve runs beside the phrenic nerve forming a reversed V towards the posterior edge of the hilum. At the thoracic inlet the pulsation of the brachiocephalic trunk or subclavian artery can be recognized. In a more dorsal direction, the oesophagus is located in the upper third of the thoracic cavity. This runs in front of the spinal column and is embedded in

Fig. 1. Thoracoscopic view of the right thoracic cavity: anatomy [21]

Fig. 2. Course of the right lung fissures in relation to the ribs

Fig. 3. Superior view
of the recess

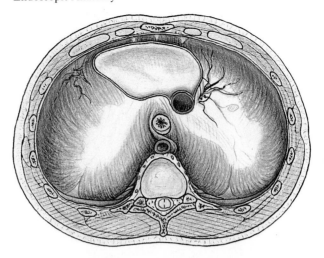

the mediastinum and covered by pleura so that it
cannot be seen thoracoscopically.

The spinal column, the costovertebral joints
and the ribs can be seen more or less clearly
defined depending on the fat content of the endothoracic fascia. At approximately the height of
the fourth rib, the azygos vein terminates in the
superior vena cava, which carries the return flow
from the intercostal veins. At the height of the
heads of the ribs, these cross the sympathetic
trunk, which can be seen clearly in thin people
and can be felt as a firm, elastic cord in all others.
From about the height of the head of the fifth
rib (sixth to ninth thoracic ganglion) the greater
splanchnic nerve arises as a sympathetic branch,
and from the height of the seventh rib (tenth
to twelfth thoracic ganglion) the lesser splanchnic
nerve arises to join the solar plexus. The sympathetic ganglia are connected to the intercostal
nerves via two to three rami communicantes. The
first ganglion (ganglion stellatum) is fused with
the last neck ganglion. This must under no circumstances be injured during thoracoscopy, since
this would cause Horner's syndrome. Ventral
to the mediastinum, the retrosternal internal
mammary artery and vein can be located and
followed easily.

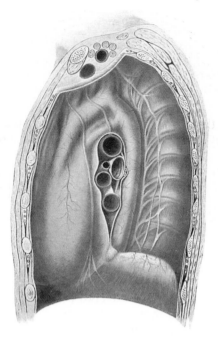

Fig. 4. Thoracoscopic view of the left thoracic cavity: anatomy [21]

The thoracic cavity forms several recesses on both sides (Fig. 3). These are important particularly with regard to inflammatory processes and when evacuating effusions or a haematoma. The most important of these is the costodiaphragmatic recess, which begins in the paravertebral region and continues in a ventral direction to become the phrenicomediastinal recess. The thoracic wall or costal pleura forms the costomediastinal recess with the mediastinum. The floor of the thoracic cavity is formed by the diaphragm. This consists of muscle and the central tendon and is also covered by pleura.

Left Thoracic Cavity [6, 10, 71, 158] (Fig. 4)
On the left-hand side, the exploration is performed in a clockwise direction. The left lung, consisting of a superior and inferior lobe only, has the oblique fissure running from dorsocranial to ventrocaudal. The lingula can nevertheless resemble a "middle lobe" when it is almost completely separate from the superior lobe, as is sometimes found.

After locating the hilum with the telescope, the phrenic nerve can once again be seen on the pericardium. This runs from cranial along the common carotid artery over the aortic arch and pericardium to the diaphragm. Lateral to the common carotid artery, the left subclavian artery arises from the aortic arch. The vagus nerve runs between these two vessels and crosses the aorta, which it then follows closely in a caudal direction. The branching of the recurrent laryngeal nerve from the vagus can sometimes be seen and often felt at the inferior edge of the aorta. The left-sided hemiazygos vein is significantly thinner than the azygos vein. It runs lateral to the aorta in a cranial direction and crosses the subclavian and carotid arteries as the accessory hemiazygos vein to terminate in the left brachiocephalic vein.

The remaining parts of the cavity are the same as those of the right-hand side.

3 Operative Technique

3.1 Instrument Set

From the point of view of performing minimally invasive interventions, the thorax and abdomen differ considerably in several aspects. The chest cavity is formed by a bony cage, which lends it stability but also makes it rigid and inflexible. The choice of entry sites for thoracoscopy is restricted by broad bones (sternum, scapulae) and the ribs and narrowed down by areas of varying muscle thickness. Owing to this bony framework, the instruments and telescopes cannot be manoeuvred freely even in areas with less musculature. Bearing in mind that the functional residual capacity of a human lung during normal breathing is 31 [69], it becomes clear that, contrary to the impression gained when the chest is open for thoracotomy, a closed chest cavity is very much smaller than the abdominal cavity. To compensate for this, intrathoracic organs are less susceptible to individual and position-dependent displacement than is the case in the abdomen. Moreover, some of the anatomical structures along the thorax wall or of the mediastinum are fixed in position and are therefore easily accessible with endoscopic techniques. Examples of such structures include the parietal pleura, the pericardium or the sympathetic trunk.

The instruments used must allow a tangential approach and be strong enough to withstand and overcome the resistance presented by the ribs. The disadvantages of the fixed pivoting point or centre of rotation can also be offset by using instruments with angled tips. With an adequately stable and rigid sheath, tactile sensitivity can also be transposed to the site of dissection.

The intercostal space limits the diameter of the trocar sleeves that can be used. Boutin et al. [21] addressed this problem several years ago and came to the conclusion that 7 mm was the ideal diameter for trocar sleeves. Larger sleeves cause pain through the periosteum of the ribs and become increasingly difficult to manoeuvre in the intercostal space; smaller sleeves do not permit the use of telescopes with adequate light intensity.

On the basis of our own studies in the thoracic cavities of cadavers, we determined the average sheath length required, the angle of the instrument tips and the diameter and necessary rigidity of the instruments. Our instrument set (Fig. 5a) was developed in conjunction with the Richard Wolf company, Germany. All instruments are available with a straight working section or angled at 25°. Apart from flexible trocar sleeves of polytetrafluoroethylene (PTFE) for introducing the instruments, rigid trocar sleeves with a lateral tap for insufflating gas and liquids are also used. All the trocar sleeves have a diameter of 7 mm to allow instruments and telescopes to be exchanged freely. The trocar tips are blunt to avoid injury to the intercostal nerves and vessels.

Other instruments are illustrated in Fig. 5b–e. The main uses of the instruments are listed in Table 1. At this point, it must be emphasized that apart from the endoscopic instruments, a thoracotomy set must be available in the theatre at all times and should therefore be considered part of thoracoscopy instrument set.

As optics (Fig. 6), we use the 7-mm straight-viewing telescope (0°) and 7-mm side-viewing 25° telescope. Side-viewing instruments with angles of view of 50° and 90° are seldom used since they complicate the co-ordinated handling of the various instruments. Moreover, with the patient in the lateral position, the 0° or 25° telescope inserted at the anterior edge of the latissimus dorsi muscle in the fourth intercostal space provides a complete overview. Depending on the distance between the telescope and the anatomical structure, a magnification factor of between 2 and 5 is possible.

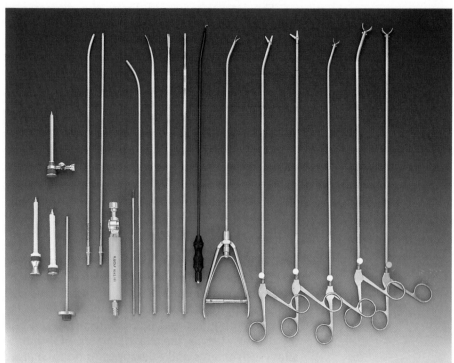

5a

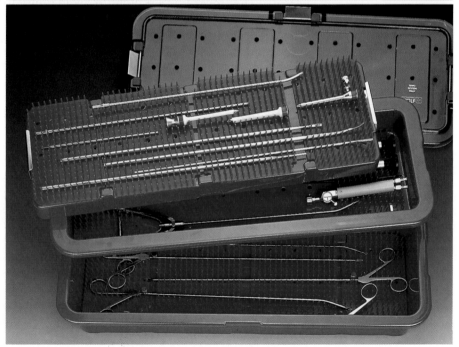

5b

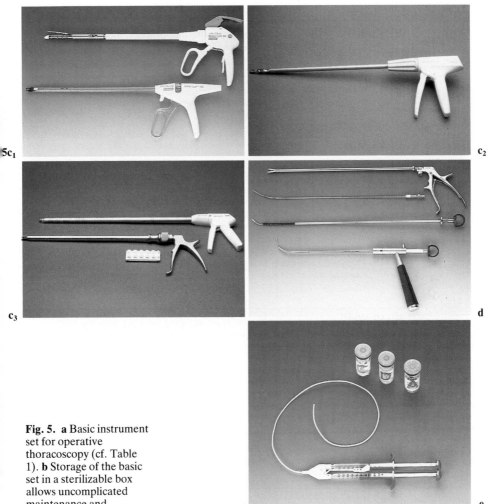

Fig. 5. **a** Basic instrument set for operative thoracoscopy (cf. Table 1). **b** Storage of the basic set in a sterilizable box allows uncomplicated maintenance and instrument care.
c Further instruments: Endo-GIA 30 stapler and endoclip applicators.
d Further instruments: Curved puncture cannula, suturing instrument with curved sharp eye, guide for sharp curved needles.
e Fibrin glue: fast and slow acting components; double lumen catheter for endoscopic application

Fig. 6. Telescopes, connector and camera (in sterile plastic bag)

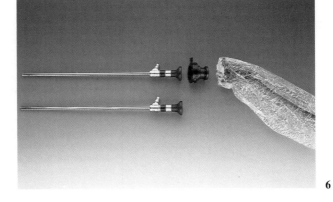

Table 1. Possible applications of thoracoscopy instruments

8243.901	Palpator: palpation, probing, measuring, adhesiolysis
8243.501 8243.502	Dissectors: palpation, adhesiolysis, dissection of tissue, débridement, decortication
8243.401 8243.402	Scissors: dividing various types of tissue (lung, pleural, mediastinum), cutting vessels, nerves and adhesions as well as suture material
8243.601 8243.602	Parenchyma grasping forceps: grasping lung parenchyma, pleura, fibrin deposits, pannus etc.
8242.202	Micro grasping forceps: grasping pleura, sympathetic trunk etc.
8242.111 8242.112	Suction/irrigation tube: suction, irrigation, débridement, decortication, adhesiolysis, palpation
8242.301	Hook electrode: coagulation, incision, dissection, adhesiolysis
8242.451	Needle holder: to guide needles, knotting, positioning Roeder loops, guiding double-lumen catheter for fibrin application

Table 1. Continued

8242.951	Guide rod: guiding and placing chest tubes
ETHIBINDER	Roeder loop: ligature of blebs and bullae and lung tissue in non-infectious fistulas or for biopsy
	Endostapler: wedge resection for pulmonary leaks, tumours, biopsy and for pericardial and cyst fenestration
	Clip applicator: haemostasis, marking
	Shaver: débridement, evacuation of fibrin deposits, dissected lung cortex, pannus, haematoma
	Injection cannula: puncture, aspiration, instillation of fibrin etc.
	Evacuation bag: for retrieving specimens
	Instrument for guiding sharp, bent needles, extendable
	Curved, sharp-tipped instrument with eye for placing ligatures, extendable

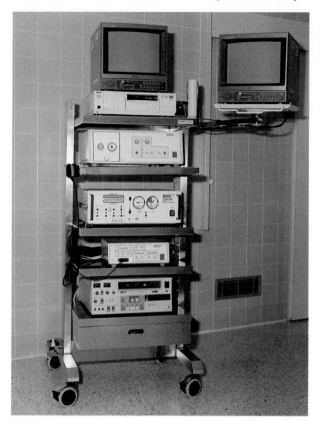

Fig. 7. Electronic devices (from top to bottom): monitors, video printer, xenon light source, endopneumothorax unit, camera, video recorder on universal video trolley

After clinical evaluation, we consider 4-mm telescopes to be unsuitable for thoracic surgery owing to the inadequate illumination they provide. Fibrescopes have also been used for thoracoscopic purposes for some time [9, 68, 155]. Comparative studies, however, came to the conclusion that rigid telescopes are easier to handle and more versatile and are therefore more suitable for thoracoscopy [115, 125]. The use of rigid scopes in minimally invasive surgery of the thoracic cavity can be considered standard. The additional intra-operative use of flexible scopes, for example to explore the pericardium (cf. Chap 16), might be of some benefit.

A charge-coupled device (CCD) chip camera is used to transmit the image to a monitor (Fig.

7). A telescope connector (Fig. 6) fitted to the camera under sterile conditions during the preparations for the intervention allows the endoscopes to be exchanged intraoperatively. We do not sterilize the video camera itself, but wrap it in a sterile, specially designed plastic cover which is commercially available.

3.2 The Operating Team

Thoracoscopic surgery, like conventional surgery, depends on teamwork. In general, one assistant in addition to the operator is adequate. It is an advantage if the assistant also has experience of endoscopic surgery and knowledge of classical surgery. With this background he is ideally suited to serve as the "cameraman", guiding the telescope, following each step of the procedure and ensuring that the operating site is in the centre of the image and in focus at all times. With his free hand the assistant can, if necessary, operate the holding forceps. Occasionally further help may be needed to apply tension to tissue or to hold tissue away from the operating site. When changing instruments, the operator or assistant steadies the trocar sleeves himself.

An anaesthetist is present whenever we perform thoracoscopy. If the intervention is performed under local anaesthesia, the anaesthetist is not only responsible for monitoring cardiorespiratory function and for administering analgesics and sedatives, but also for the intraoperative psychological welfare of the patient. To fulfil this function, the anaesthetist must be fully informed about the planned operation in advance.

Well-practised teamwork is also essential when the patient is under general anaesthesia to ensure efficient double-lumen intubation (cf. Sect. 3.6).

Care and maintenance of the instruments, some of which are particularly delicate, and suitable storage of the instrument sets, making them readily available at all times, demands highly motivated staff. For the operation to run smoothly, staff must be thoroughly familiar with the instrument set, the electronic units and the wide variety of accessories. The instrumentation team will take a greater interest in minimally invasive surgery if they are fully informed about the purpose of the operation and are directly involved in the events taking place. The instrument nurse should also be able to follow the operation on the monitor (cf. Sect. 3.4).

The tasks undertaken by the circulating nurse are just as important. The settings of the video camera, the high-performance light source and the insufflation unit must be adapted regularly to the current intraoperative situation. For example, even minor bleeding absorbs light, whereas shiny instruments can reflect so much light that the automatic light regulation reduces the brightness. The degree of suction of the aspirator must also be adjusted, and irrigation solution containers topped up. Additional equipment such as suturing materials and fibrin glue must be placed at hand so that they can be brought to the operating table quickly. Operation of the recording devices (video recorder, photoprinter, stills camera) is also important.

This demands not only that the surgeon instructs staff thoroughly, but also the recognition that a successful thoracoscopy is not dependent on the operator alone but is the result of well coordinated teamwork.

3.3 Preparing the Patient

Admission Assessment
The admission of a patient for thoracoscopy does not differ in any way from the normal procedure for surgical patients. A comprehensive medical history is obtained and the clinical examinations performed and documented thoroughly and carefully. Radiological examinations, laboratory tests and preoperative examinations are performed according to the clinical findings.

Particular attention is paid to possible causes of pleural obliteration in order to be able to select the best patient position and most promising sites of entry or to avoid an unnecessary attempt at thoracoscopy. If the medical history and the clinical and conventional radiological findings are clear, computed tomography can often be helpful, since even slight thickening of the pleura and differences between the two sides can be recognized (Fig. 8).

Patient Interview

Since minimally invasive surgery mainly involves new techniques for which no reliable long-term results are yet available, the patient must be thoroughly informed about the intended operation and the alternatives in such a way that he or she understands the situation. The patient must be aware that while the visible entry site is smaller than the normal surgical incision, the technique nevertheless involves internal wound surfaces just as in any surgical intervention and that these can mean a deterioration in general condition and cause pain. The patient must also understand that converting the intervention to a thoracotomy intraoperatively is not necessarily the result of a complication, but must be considered as a planned eventuality if the situation exceeds the possibilities of endoscopic techniques. In this context, the surgeon should also explain that a thoracoscopy begun under local anaesthesia may

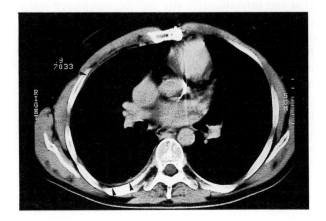

Fig. 8. CT scan showing slight thickening of the pleura: ventral and paraventral on the right side various areas of more extensive thickening visible (arrows). These areas, which cannot be recognized on conventional X-ray films, are important for preoperative planning of the incisions

have to be continued under general intubation
anaesthesia.

The drainage tubes protruding from the chest
often frighten patients and inhibit their whole-
hearted support of physiotherapeutic measures intended to restore mobility as quickly as possible.
For this reason, they should be informed preoperatively both of the purpose of drains and
of the physiotherapeutic strategies for preventing
thrombosis and atelectasis; this will clarify in the
patient's mind the need to perform postoperative
exercises despite pain.

The aim of such a discussion should be to
build up a rapport with the patient. Gaining
the patient's trust and conveying to him that his
worries and questions are being taken seriously is
a fundamental part of a surgeon's job and involves
far more than simply obtaining a signature on the
consent form.

Preoperative Examinations
The normal sequence of preoperative examinations is listed in Table 2. Whether or not a particular examination is performed depends on the
indications and the possible clinical relevance of
the examination.

3.4 Patient Positioning

The patient lies on a radiolucent operating table.
Even though this is seldom necessary, it ensures
that the intrathoracic site can be visualized intraoperatively with an image intensifier.

The patient position and theatre arrangement
must allow the operating team to work comfortably and without physical stress. The sterile drapes
must be arranged so that a thoracotomy can be
performed quickly and unhindered. Two positions
have proved to be suitable.

Table 2. Preoperative evaluation

Anamnesis
  Search for indications of pleural obliteration
    Previous operations?
    Condition following irradiation?
    Pulmonary tuberculosis, bouts of pneumonia?
  Indications of pleural conditions
    Exposure to asbestos
    Neoplasia
    Drugs
  Chronic pulmonary disease
    Chronic obstructive pneumopathy
    Bronchial asthma
    Others
  Current medication
    Steroids
    Immunosuppressants
    Drugs affecting clotting

Clinical examination
  Inspection of the posture and configuration of the thorax
  Respiratory symmetry; degree of thorax musculature, scars
  Percussion and auscultation, particularly margins of the diaphragm and mobility
  Mobility of shoulders (both shoulders with a view to positioning on table)

Laboratory tests
  Haemoglobin, thrombocytes, prothrombin times, international normalized ratio
  Analysis of pleural effusions: protein, lactate dehydrogenase, glucose, pH; amylase,
  triglyceride, cytology; microbiology

Imaging techniques
  Chest X-ray, AP and lateral views
  Depending on anamnesis, findings and clinical questions
    Computed tomography
    Sonography, transthoracic and/or transoesophageal

Pulmonary function tests
  The indication depends on the anamnesis, the clinical findings and the planned
  thoracoscopic intervention

Cardiological examination
  The necessity of this depends on the anamnesis, the clinical findings and the planned
  thoracoscopic intervention.
    ECG with/without rhythm strips
    Further cardiological examinations

Lateral Position (Fig. 9)

Analogous to open thoracic surgery, the lateral position can be considered standard. Via the access sites described, this position allows a complete view of the thoracic cavity, and all types of interventions attempted up to now can be performed with optimum efficiency. Care must be taken to ensure that the upper arm on the operation side does not extend above shoulder level, since this would hinder the manoeuvrability of the instruments and telescopes in the cranial direction and restrict the view and manipulations in the basal areas of the thoracic cavity.

Supine Position (Fig. 10)

The supine position is suitable (a) for interventions under local infiltration anaesthesia, (b) when a patient's general condition would not allow a prolonged lateral position, (c) when the possibility of a change to anaesthesia by endotracheal intubation during the operation cannot be excluded.

Other Positions

Other positions are possible but seldom used. Examples include the lateral (semi-prone) position for paravertebral evacuation of an encapsulated liquid mass (cf. Sect. 12) or the semi-sitting position for performing pleurodesis in cases of malignant pleural effusion in cachectic patients with marginal respiratory reserves (cf. Sect. 17).

Sterile Drapes

The most successful drape has proved to be a large, disposable U-shaped split-window drape with self-adhesive edges. At shoulder height, a second self-adhesive drape is positioned at right angles to the first drape. The metal anaesthesia screen at the patient's head is positioned as far cephalad as possible to allow the unobstructed movement of instruments and telescopes in the sagittal plane above shoulder level. This draping arrangement demands a certain "give and take" on the part of the surgeon and anaesthetist.

Fig. 9. Standard position: patient in lateral position. On the side to be operated on, the upper arm must not extend above the shoulder to prevent movement of the telescopes and instruments being obstructed

Fig. 10. Patient in supine position

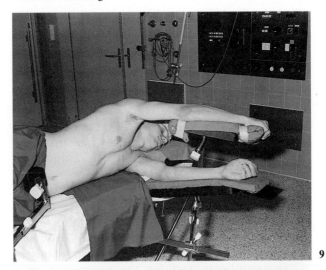

9

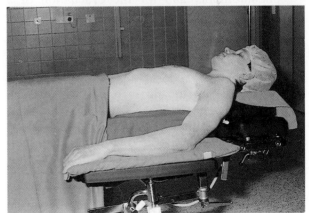

10

3.5 Anaesthesia

Anaesthesia plays a major role in thoracoscopic surgery. The suitable choice of anaesthesia and adequate alleviation of pain are decisive factors influencing the patient's fast recovery and his or her psychological and physical reintegration. Suitable anaesthesia and the preoperative talk with the patient can reduce anxiety and stress.

We use the following three techniques of anaesthesia:

1. Local infiltration anaesthesia: this method is used with the patient's consent in purely diagnostic thoracoscopy when adhesions are not expected, in cases of idiopathic spontaneous pneumothorax and for the evacuation of a haematoma before it becomes organized. Low doses of sedatives and intravenous painkillers are nevertheless often necessary with these indications. The incision sites are anaesthetized with 10 ml of a local anaesthetic 1% (e.g. Xylocaine) up to and including the parietal pleura. Each sensitive structure (the skin, periosteum, intercostal nerve and parietal pleura) must be located and injected individually. Some authors use an adrenalin additive to prevent blood from seeping into the incision [21]. This is intended to prevent blood running along the trocar sleeve and obscuring the view through the scope.

    With this method of anaesthesia the patient must be thoroughly informed prior to the operation and must receive suitable psychological support during the operation. The anaesthetist can communicate with the conscious patient allowing thorough anaesthesiological monitoring. Compared with intubation anaesthesia, the physiological strain on the patient during the operation is also reduced. A contraindication to the use of local anaesthesia is allergic reaction to the required drugs.
2. Local anaesthesia combined with neuroleptanalgesia: the additional neuroleptic agent is

administered i.v. either as premedication before the patient is positioned or during the intervention. The indications correspond to those for local infiltration anaesthesia. The substances used should combine adequate sedation with an anxiolytic effect. An additional amnesic effect is desirable during longer interventions with consequent pain resulting from the patient position.

3. Endotracheal intubation with a double-lumen tube: this is the method we use most commonly. In nervous patients it must also be used when local anaesthesia would otherwise be indicated. The major advantage of this method compared with others is that it allows an operation on the "open thorax", i.e. after induction of the pneumothorax and collapsing the lobe of the lung, the operation can continue without further gas insufflation and with the trocar sleeves left open. Endoscopes and instruments can be removed and repositioned as necessary. Generally, we ventilate the collapsed lung for 3 min every 20 min to prevent atelectasis, shunt problems and pulmonary vasoconstriction.

Single endotracheal intubation is a compromise solution when a double-lumen tube cannot be introduced for technical reasons. It should, when possible, be avoided. The advantages of the collapsed lung and the reduced invasiveness of the local anaesthesia are lost. If this technique is, however, used, the anaesthesiological technique should allow the patient to breathe spontaneously. In this way, at least a partial pneumothorax without ventilatory counter-pressure can be maintained as under local anaesthesia.

The routine techniques used by our anaesthetists are explained in Table 3. The intraoperative monitoring of the patient is described in Table 4.

The choice of anaesthetic technique depends on the patient, the indications and the planned intervention. The experience of the surgeon and anaesthetist can also be a deciding factor. As a

Table 3. Anaesthesia techniques

Local infiltration anaesthesia

Premedication:
Oral administration of a mild anxiolytic/sedative of the diazepam group, combined with an opioid (e.g. nicomorphine hydrochloride)

Infiltration anaesthesia
Each entry site is rendered insensitive with 10 ml of a 1% local anaesthetic (e.g. Scandicain) without adrenaline

Intravenous analgesia/sedation

Premedication:
Oral administration of a mild anxiolytic/sedative of the diazepam group, combined with an opioid (e.g. nicomorphine hydrochloride)

Intraoperative
1. Opioid with short duration of action, e.g. alfentanil. If necessary the substance can be administered several times
2. Propofol. This is infused while clinically monitoring the parameters listed in Table 4 or is injected continuously using a perfusor in longer interventions
3. Each entry site is rendered insensitive with 10 ml of a 1% local anaesthetic (e.g. Scandicain) without adrenaline

Intubation anaesthesia using the double-lumen technique

Premedication
Oral administration of a mild anxiolytic/sedative of the diazepam group, possibly combined with an opioid (e.g. nicomorphine hydrochloride)

Induction of anaesthesia
1. Rapid-acting barbiturate, e.g. thiopentone
2. Rapid-acting, depolarizing muscle relaxant, e.g. succinylcholine

Maintenance of anaesthesia
1. N_2O/O_2, insufflation at a ratio 4:2 (pulse oximetry monitoring!) With single lung anaesthesia: N_2O/O_2 ratio 1:1
2. Non-depolarizing, rapid-acting muscle relaxant, e.g. atracurium
3. Opioid with short duration of action, e.g. alfentanil

Table 4. Intraoperative monitoring of the thoracoscopy patient

---

All forms of anaesthesia
  Continuous electrocardiography
  Regular measurement of blood pressure with upper arm
    cuff
  Continuous transcutaneous measurement of oxygen
    saturation (Biox)

Additionally for intubation anaesthesia
  Continuous measurement of CO_2 content in expired breath
    (capnography)

---

rule of thumb: if in doubt, use double-lumen intubation.

The possible complications during anaesthesia correspond to those encountered in open lung surgery. With the exception of those patients who were already being artificially ventilated prior to surgery ($n = 3$), all patients ($n = 247$) could be extubated immediately following the operation.

The literature includes reports of, in some cases, considerable numbers of patients experiencing postoperative nausea and vomiting after laparoscopic surgery [29, 79]. We did not observe this in our patients. We recall two patients with some degree of postoperative nausea, in one of which this cleared up very quickly as soon as we discontinued giving a morphine derivative to alleviate pain.

3.6 Inducing the Pneumothorax

To perform thoracoscopy we induce a pneumothorax. Possible obliteration should be searched for preoperatively (cf. Sect. 3.3). With increasing experience, both the preoperative localization of possible pleural adhesions and the recognition of a completely obliterated pleural space becomes easier. During the first 50 thoracoscopies we performed, we had to discontinue the intervention in 6% of cases owing to obliteration; since then this has only been necessary in 1.5% of more than 180 operations.

For a better understanding of the pneumothorax, a brief outline of the physiology of the pleural space should be helpful. At the mid-height of the pleural space in minute respiration at rest and with the body in an upright position, there is a negative pressure of -0.4 to $-0.5\,$kPa. At the base of the lung, the negative pressure is approximately $-0.3\,$kPa less, at $-0.2\,$kPa, whereas at the apex it is approximately $-1.0\,$kPa. Deeper inspiration generally results in a higher negative pressure, since the elastic retraction forces of the lung increase. At maximum expansion of the lung these values can rise to $-40\,$cm H_2O. Deep exhalation results in values around 0 or slightly positive. The difference in intrapleural pressure between the base of the lung and the apex of $-0.7\,$kPa remains unchanged in all inspiratory and expiratory phases [184].

For operative thoracoscopy, it is an advantage to induce an extended pneumothorax, although this is not always necessary. The degree of collapse of the lung required to perform the intervention depends on how well the structure involved can be visualized.

To induce the pneumothorax we use an endopneu insufflator, familiar from laparoscopy. With the commonly used insufflation units, the insufflation pressure can be set and measured in mmHg at any time. The quality of the gas flow (laminar

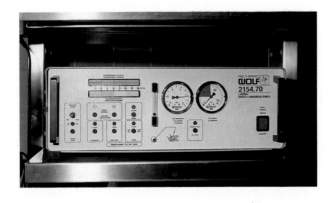

Fig. 11. Endoscopic insufflation unit with pressure limiting function, flow glass, flowmeter and CO_2 cylinder content indicator (from left to right)

or turbulent) can also be checked. Finally, the required flow per minute can be selected (Fig. 11). CO_2 is used for safety reasons owing to its fast reabsorption if gas is accidentally forced into extrapleural, and in particular vascular or mediastinal structures.

We consider the use of the endo-insufflator an advantage for a further practical reason. If only the natural pleural negative pressure is used to induce the pneumothorax when the thorax is opened, a partial pneumothorax is formed, which is seldom adequate for thorough exploration of the whole pleural space. The CO_2 insufflation, which is continued under vision after the initial 500 ml, allows controlled, but fast deflation of the lung without reducing the safety provided by the endo-insufflator functions listed above. As an alternative, a pneumothorax unit can be used, as found commonly in pneumology [21, 26].

In a small study of the intrapleural pressures when using the endo insufflator involving ten patients, we discovered that during insufflation of CO_2 at a preselected rate of 1 l/m and with the maximum pressure limited to 15 mmHg, the intrapleural pressure in the initial phase of the pneumothorax varied between -2 and $+1$ cm H_2O. When operating under local anaesthesia or endotracheal intubation anaesthesia without a doublelumen tube, i.e. with a closed pneumothorax system, pressure peaks of up to $+15$ cm H_2O were registered during attacks of coughing. With a non-ventilated lung and double-lumen intubation, on the other hand, the intrapleural pressure with the lung collapsed and the trocar sleeves open was, as might be expected, ambient pressure. The study was performed using a unit which records the intrapleural pressure in cm H_2O by means of an electronic transducer.

The first incision, standardly made at the highest point anterior to the latissimus dorsi muscle (cf. Fig. 16), is used to introduce the Verres needle if a free thoracic cavity is expected. When the pleural space is punctured with the Verres needle, its position is checked in three ways. As the needle passes into the pleural space, the operator both feels and hears a slight "pop-ping". The slurp test is performed by filling the Verres needle with Ringer's solution. If the tip of the needle passes through the parietal pleura unobstructed, the drop of water sitting on the top of the needle is sucked in by the negative in-trathoracic pressure. After connecting the needle to the pneumothorax unit via a plastic tube, the CO_2 gas is insufflated while checking the direct flow indicator and the preselected insufflation pressure. If the flow is unobstructed, approxi-mately 500 ml of CO_2 are insufflated initially. In a pleural space free of adhesions, the negative intrapleural pressure sucks the gas in through the needle, so that the displayed insufflation pres-sure only exceeds 2–4 mmHg on the scale during spontaneous forced inspiration with the patient under local anaesthesia. A higher pressure indica-tion and a slow flow rate suggest a septate pleural space caused by adhesions, partial obliteration, or incorrect positioning of the needle with its tip in the thoracic wall. If, on the other hand, the capnograph indicates a rise in the expired CO_2 corresponding to the gas insufflation, the Verres needle is most probably in the lung parenchyma and must be repositioned.

If it proves impossible to induce a pneumo-thorax, a mini-incision can be made to allow local digital palpation of the pleural cavity before deciding whether to discontinue or to perform a thoracotomy. With his fingers, an experienced surgeon will be able to distinguish between an old and/or thick band and delicate adhesions or fresh, currently organizing pannus. In the case of the latter two findings, a circumscribed cavity can be formed with a finger. After sealing the incision with skin sutures, two trocars are inserted close to each other to allow the telescope and an in-strument (palpator or suction tube) to be intro-duced. Under optical control, the adhesions can be divided step by step and the pleural space freed. At the same time, the lung is collapsed by CO_2 insufflation. This technique is only suitable for double-lumen intubated patients.

The dangers involved in inducing the pneumothorax are gas embolism, mediastinal emphysema, generalized air emphysema and serious dyspnoea. The clinical significance of these complications is discussed in Chap. 4.

The surgeon and anaesthetist must be ready to take action if a patient under local anaesthesia becomes anxious while the pneumothorax is being induced. While the surgeon stops further gas insufflation or, if the symptoms are severe, reverses the pneumothorax, the anaesthetist assesses the clinical relevance of the situation and takes psychological and, if necessary, medical measures to allay anxiety and calm the patient. To date, we have not yet had to abandon thoracoscopy due to patient anxiety.

3.7 Drainage

Following thoracic surgery, including thoracoscopic interventions, special postoperative measures are necessary owing to the negative physiological pressure in the pleural space (cf. Sect. 3.6). There is a potential risk of pleural callosities or a residual dead space forming if air fistula or postoperative collections of fluid are inadequately drained. To avoid this, large-lumen thorax drains must be placed correctly. As routine, we insert a ventroapical air drain and a dorsoinferior fluid drain in the costodiaphragmatic recess. The drains must not be placed in the pulmonary fissures since they draw in the lung parenchyma and cease to function.

The drainage should cause a negative intrapleural pressure to re-establish normal physiological conditions as quickly as possible. The successful re-establishment of physiological conditions with a pleural space free of fluid and air can be confirmed radiologically by the normal anatomical position of the mediastinum, the convexity of the diaphragm and symmetrical intercostal spaces. The normal expansion of the lung can be recognized by the absence of atelectasis and dystelectasis.

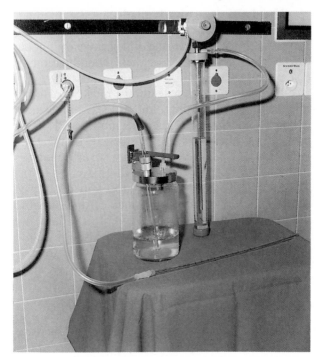

Fig. 12. Thoracic drainage system. Thoracic drain, bottle and water seal

The simplest form of pleural drainage system is to seal the extension of the tube by water in a bottle. The bottle must be lower than the patient. This produces a vacuum of between -3 and -5 mmHg. To achieve a faster expansion of the lung when a larger volume of fluid or an air fistula is involved, continuous suction can be applied to the system (Fig. 12). The strength of the suction applied should be such that the increasing negative intrapleural pressure is exceeded during inspiration. If the pleural secretion in the system moves towards the patient during inspiration, this is not the case.

The intermittent formation of bubbles in the water seal also indicates insufficient suction or a large leak in the lung. If, despite continuous suction and the absence of bubbles, the water level in the tubing moves backwards and forwards between the thorax wall and the bottle, this suggests an established dead space or trapped lung.

Fig. 13. Types of
drainage tubes: straight
and curved thoracic
tubes, 20–30 Fr.,
"Mathy" chest tube

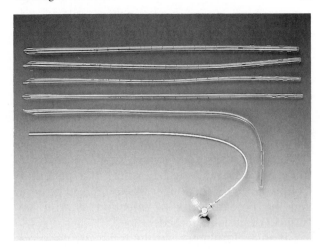

A thorax drain should not be clamped! This
avoids the risk of a tension pneumothorax, and
the desired adhesion between the lung and thorax
wall is not broken. The water-filled bottle must,
however, not be raised higher than the patient.
The nursing staff must be appropriately instructed
and informed of the reasons for this. In this context, daily inquiries by the surgeon about the
amount and type of secretion and a personal check
of the apparatus should be part of the postoperative management. The patient should be informed about the purpose of the thorax drainage
prior to the intervention (cf. Sect. 3.3).

The tubes used should always have a large
diameter. Figure 13 shows the types of drain used
in our department. The choice of type, number
and length of the intrathoracic section depend on
the intervention performed and the anatomical –
pathological situation. The exit sites of the tubes
should not be in the area of the patient's back nor
in the axilla to achieve optimum drainage and to
reduce patient discomfort. We usually use two
of the three entry sites as exits for the drains.
Effectiveness takes priority over cosmesis and
comfort.

If clinical and radiological examination shows
the lung to be expanded, no more air is escaping
via the drain and the amount of secretion is below

100 ml of clear serous fluid in 24 h (approximately the amount of secretion resulting from the irritation caused by the drain itself), the drain is removed. Following short thoracoscopies under local anaesthesia where no large-scale surgery was undertaken, we ignore the amount of secretion. The drain is removed, ideally in the inspiratory position to avoid a sudden reflex inspiration by the patient.

Leaving the drain longer than necessary is therapeutically undesirable, since the patient is troubled by pain the longer the drain is in position and the potential risk of infection as with any surgical drain is increased.

If an air fistula persists the following questions must be clarified:

–   Is the drainage system between the vacuum connection and thorax drain blocked, is there a leak, is part of the system disconnected? (Clinical check required.)
–   Is the drain entry site into the thorax airtight? (Clinical check required.)
–   Has the drain become loose in the holding suture and partly slipped out? Are there lateral openings in the drain outside the thoracic cavity? (Radiological check required.)
–   Is the intrathoracic section correctly positioned? (When placing the drain intraoperatively, the displacement of the tip by the expansion of the lung must be taken into consideration.)
–   Is the thoracoscopically applied ligature, the staple suture or the applied fibrin airtight? (Review of the video tape of the operation, if necessary second-look thoracoscopy.)
–   Is the suspected air fistula infected or is it close to a tumour? (Review of the video tape of the operation, if necessary second-look thoracoscopy or thoracotomy (cf. Chap. 13).)

Correctly placed tubes, adequate suction and competent postoperative handling of the drainage system are decisive for the success of thoracoscopic interventions.

Fig. 14. Arrangement in
the operating theatre with
the patient in the lateral
position

Fig. 15. Arrangement in
the operating theatre with
the patient in the supine
position

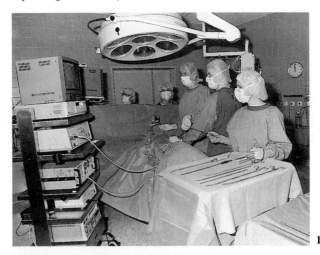

14

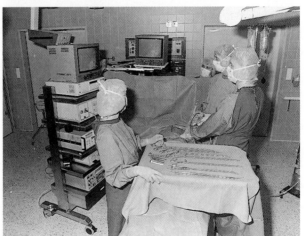

15

3.8 Operating Theatre Layout

If the operation is performed with the patient in
the lateral position, the surgeon, assistant and
theatre sister stand ventral to the patient. The unit
trolley with the TV monitor is positioned on the
opposite side at the height of the thorax (Fig. 14).

If the intervention is performed with the
patient in the supine position, the whole team
stands on the side of the patient on which the
operation will take place with the monitor on the

opposite side. By positioning the theatre nurse on the same side as the operating team, she can also view the screen and can actively participate in the operation, improving co-operation. If a second monitor is installed, the nurse can also stand on the opposite side. This creates more space and further improves efficiency (Fig. 15).

An adequately large room in which the various devices can be installed comfortably is certainly desirable. When installing the assortment of cables and tubes leading into the sterile field, space must be left to ensure unobstructed access to the various units (video unit, insufflator, coagulation unit, suction apparatus, etc.). We prefer a star-shaped arrangement of all the equipment.

3.9 Incision Sites

When selecting the incision sites, bony structures in the thorax (ribs, sternum and scapula), muscular regions (greater and smaller pectoral muscles, latissimus dorsi and anterior serratus muscles) nerves (long thoracic and thoracodorsal nerves) and intercostal blood vessels must be taken into account. The incisions should be selected so that vessels and nerves are not injured and the telescope and instruments can be manoeuvred freely.

Depending on the planned surgery and position of pathological findings, the incisions are made between the third and eighth intercostal spaces. Once again, it must not be forgotten that in the area of the inlet of the thorax there is little space between the wall of the chest and the mediastinum with its large vessels, and the instruments must be introduced slowly and carefully. In the basal regions of the thorax, it is not unusual for the phrenicocostal sinus to be scarred following pleuritis and elevated in a cranial direction and there is the risk of penetrating the liver or spleen if the trocar is not inserted carefully.

In the technique we found most suitable, three mini-incisions are made in the non-muscular axillary triangle formed by the axilla, the posterior

Fig. 16. Standard entry
sites in lateral position

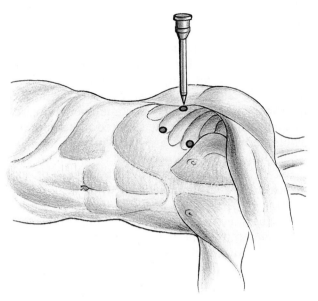

edge of the greater pectoral muscle and the
anterior edge of the latissimus dorsi muscle (Fig.
16). In the lateral position, the first incision is
always made anterior to the latissimus dorsi muscle in the fourth intercostal space and in the
supine position at the posterior edge of the greater
pectoral muscle at the height of the fifth intercostal space. With the double-lumen tube in
place, the ventilation of the lung involved is
first discontinued. After inserting a rigid trocar
through the skin incision, the CO_2 tube is connected to the lateral trocar tap. The straight-
viewing telescope is then introduced. All the
endoscopic manoeuvres are now transmitted to a
colour monitor. To complete the pneumothorax,
further CO_2 is insufflated.

The second and third incisions form a triangle
and are made at sufficient distance from each
other in the area between the second and eighth
intercostal spaces. The position of the access sites
is decided depending on the operation and can
now be verified or modified as result of the visual
inspection. Normally only the skin is incised.
We use flexible PTFE trocars with a diameter

of 7 mm. The blunt, conical tip helps to avoid injuries to the intercostal vessels and lungs. If sail-like adhesions are found (Fig. 17), which can prevent the insertion of trocars under optical control, probing with a fine needle mounted on a syringe filled with saline or fluoroscopy with the image intensifier used as routine by some pneumologists [26] may show whether the selected route of entry would terminate in a gas-filled pleural area or would injure lung parenchyma.

A "Z" technique through the layers of the thorax wall, as commonly used when introducing a drain, has proved of no value in thoracoscopy. The subcutaneous tunnelling and final transmuscular penetration in the next higher intercostal space would stretch the skin and further hinder the free movement of the instruments in the trocar sleeve already restricted by the fixed pivoting point in the intercostal space.

Blood seeping from the puncture channel tends to run along the trocar sleeve to its inner opening. When the telescope is introduced, the view through the window is obscured. This can be prevented firstly by blunt penetration of the thoracic wall, secondly by applying an anti-misting agent to the window, thirdly by rinsing the trocar sleeve with Ringer's solution or cleaning it through

Fig. 17. a Endoscopic image: elastic sail-like adhesions. In the lower part of the figure lung parenchyma can be seen, and *at the top* the thorax wall. These adhesions obstruct the induction of a pneumothorax. b If the Verres needle is inserted at a point with such adhesions between the lung and wall of the chest, there is a danger of the tip penetrating lung parenchyma. *Middle*, adhesions; *top*, thoracic wall; *bottom*, lung parenchyma

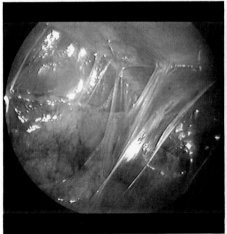

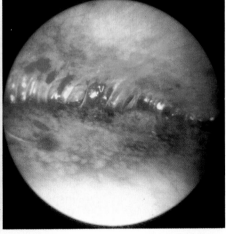

a   b

with a gauze sponge as if cleaning a gun barrel. Up to now, no ideal solution to this irritating problem has been found. Suggested solutions involving a jet on the tip of the telescope meant a reduction in diameter and intolerable loss of light. We have not observed clinically significant bleeding caused by trocars injuring intercostal vessels in the area of the incision. When this did occur, it was the result of intraoperative injury by the instruments.

3.10 General Operative Steps

After successfully establishing the entry sites, every thoracoscopic intervention begins with the exploration of the thoracic cavity. This part of the procedure should be standardized to avoid overlooking pathological findings. The exploration of the left side starts from a position anterior to the hilum and continues in clockwise direction and on the right side in an anti-clockwise direction (cf. Chap. 2). The palpator and grasping forceps are extremely useful for exposing the anatomical structures, especially in obese patients (e.g. the sympathetic trunk and the recurrent laryngeal nerve). With increasing experience the instrumental palpation provides more information about the pathological findings in terms of consistency, origin and relationship to surrounding structures (Fig. 45).

Before beginning the actual intervention, the whole thoracic cavity and its structures (including the fissures) should always be thoroughly inspected. Only then is a precise assessment possible, following which the operation can be finally planned. Overlooked or deliberately ignored adhesions create blind spots and can complicate or even prevent correct and fast instrument handling in the case of bleeding, which can appear more severe than it is owing to the endoscopic magnification.

Obstructing adhesions are divided with the scissors or monopolar coagulation probe (Fig. 17). Sharp dissection with scissors is unproblematic,

since any bleeding which does occur is almost
without exception on the parietal side of the adhesion and can be coagulated immediately.

It is now useful to introduce the suction irrigation tube. An isotonic, crystalline solution at
body temperature can then be instilled for irrigation. Only a solution at body temperature should
be used since colder fluid may lead to a vasovagal
reflex (cf. Chap. 4). The tip of the tube can
be used for dissection with the irrigation flow
activated. The water jet is also helpful in locating sources of bleeding. Whenever solution is
aspirated, CO_2 must be insufflated at the same
time or a trocar left open to prevent the lung from
expanding.

At the end of each intervention, haemostasis
must be thoroughly checked and parenchyma leaks
located if there is a possibility that the surface
of the lung has been injured. The best way of
checking for leaks is to use the "water test". The
lung is carefully ventilated and then pressed section by section below the surface of instilled
Ringer's solution using the palpator.

The drains are then placed through the existing
mini-incisions under vision and their tips positioned at the apex and in the phrenicocostal sinus
aided by the guide rod (Fig. 18). The evacuation
of the pneumothorax to complete the intervention

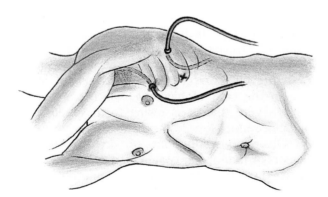

Fig. 18. The chest tubes
can often be inserted
through existing incisions
when the thoracoscopy is
complete

should be performed under optical vision and performed slowly to avoid interstitial pulmonary oedema.

The remaining incisions are closed with a single suture which can be removed after 7 days.

3.11 After-Care in the Hospital

One of the main aims of the minimally invasive technique is the conservation or the thoracic wall important for respiratory function. By precise dissection under two- to fivefold magnification, the internal wound surface can also be kept to a minimum. Whether keeping the organs in the closed thoracic cavity and thereby protecting them from drying under the glare of the operating lights has any positive effect would have to be established by taking tissue specimens for comparison.

Despite the proven and potential advantages of the technique, the patient does suffer operative trauma, even after thoracoscopy. Anaesthesia is induced, the lung is collapsed and inner wound surfaces are created. Possible results of the operation could be seen in X-rays taken routinely 24 h after the operation, which revealed one case of lobe atelectasis and several cases of dystelectasis of the parenchyma. The after-care is the same as after standard open thoracic surgery. However, the patient does not see the "obvious evidence" of the operation he or she has undergone, i.e. the thoracotomy wound. A talk prior to the operation is then all the more important to motivate the patient to co-operate actively in the postoperative phase. Intensive respiratory exercises and physiotherapy and mobilization on the day of the operation are the foundations of the postoperative care.

In our experience, whether or not the patient should be moved to a recovery room after the operation depends more on the routine of the individual hospital than on the thoracoscopic intervention performed. We generally move patients back to their department. Exceptions to this are cachectic patients with malignant effusions following pleurodesis and patients who for social or psychological reasons (e.g. addicts) are transferred to the monitoring ward in our own department.

The routine postoperative monitoring during the first few hours is carried out according to the parameters shown in Table 5. Thorax drains should not be clamped, otherwise they serve no purpose and create a false sense of security. If symptoms are unclear and a drain is in place, the differential diagnosis is unlikely to be the development of a tension pneumothorax or haemothorax (see Sect. 3.7 for drainage methods and removal of drains).

Once the anaesthesia has worn off, the majority of patients have pain during the first few hours in the side of the thorax in which the endoscopy was performed. If the pain is localized in the area of the incision, this can be attributed to traumatized periosteum, although patients rarely complain of this pain. Much more common is an undefined pain in the shoulder area, regardless of the intervention performed. This possibly reflects a diffuse pleural irritation caused by the intervention itself or by the CO_2. The latter is also described following laparoscopic surgery with a corresponding pneumoperitoneum [141]. The longer the drains are left in place, the more patients complain of discomfort and pain, which can best be alleviated by additionally taping the drain to the skin. Following the patient's instructions is the only way to find the best position.

The large number of publications concerning thoracoscopy only contain occasional references to postoperative pain. Routinely, we administer paracetamol for 48 h at a dosage of 2000 mg/24 h and, if necessary nicomorphine. The mean dosage of nicomorphine in our series was 11.5 mg/24 h. This value did not depend on the particular intervention performed.

The length of hospitalization depends on the clinical condition and social environment of the patient. If the parameters listed in Table 6 are unremarkable in the first 8 h and if the patient will be cared for at home, there is nothing to prevent discharge on the same day or after brief

Table 5. Postoperative monitoring[a]

Continuous monitoring
Electrocardiography
Transcutaneous measurement of oxygen saturation (Biox)
At brief intervals
Blood pressure
Respiratory frequency
Consciousness
Correct functioning of chest tube
Administration of 2–4 l oxygen until O_2 saturation normalizes

[a] After all forms of anaesthesia. No problems between 3 and 6 h

Table 6. Complications arising from thoracoscopy

Complications		Occurrences in 251 of our own cases
Bleeding	Arterial	3
	Venous	1
Lung parenchyma	Injury	5
	Persistent pneumothorax after biopsy (>24 h)	1
	Atelectasis	1[a]
	Pneumonia	1[a]
	Interstitial expansion oedema	1
Air emphysema	Local subcutaneous	Common
	Generalized	1[a]
	Mediastinal emphysema	1[a]
Tension pneumothorax		1
Infection	Pneumonia	2[a]
Thoracic hyp-/dysaesthesia		1
Cardiac dysrhythmia	Vasovagal reflex with bradycardia <40 beats/min	1
Postoperative fever		20%
Postoperative pain		Common

[a] One patient

hospitalization. The continuity of the follow-up must, however, be guaranteed and this gains in importance the shorter the hospital stay. The discharged patient should also be able to contact the surgeon responsible for his or her therapy at any time.

4 Dangers and Risks of the Method

Large control series reported in the considerable body of literature dealing with diagnostic and interventional thoracoscopy confirm the low mortality and morbidity of the method. Viskum [173] found only one fatality in over 8000 recorded cases. In a review of the literature by Boutin et al. [19], the mortality rate was 0.09% in more than 4300 cases. It must, however, be pointed out that these figures primarily involved conventional thoracoscopic interventions for biopsy or to perform pleurodesis in cases of malignant effusions and spontaneous pneumothorax. These interventions are normally performed under local anaesthesia combined with intravenous sedation via one and more seldom two incisions.

Within the framework of conventional thoracoscopy, the following side effects and complications have been reported: haemothorax [21, 125, 142, 172], mediastinal emphysema, subcutaneous tension emphysema and generalized air emphysema [21, 166], air embolism [49, 172], pleural empyema [21, 33, 38], re-expansion pulmonary oedema [21], injuries to the lung [21] and tumorous contamination of the incision site [21, 33, 113, 114]. In addition to these, cardiac dysrhythmia [48, 125], hypotonia [38, 70], vasovagal reactions [172] and hypoxaemia [21, 125, 172] have all been described. Reports of serious complications do, however, remain isolated cases.

Comparable statistics for operative thoracoscopy do not yet exist as far as we are aware. Conclusions based on the experience of laparoscopic surgery can be, at best, tentative. Accidental puncture of abdominal vessels caused by inserting the needle too deep or without adequate control [143] may be analogous to injury of the delicate pulmonary vessels or mediastinal veins in the thoracic cavity.

In our series, none of the 251 patients operated on between January 1990 and April 1992 died as the immediate result of thoracoscopy: nine patients died within 30 days:

– Seven cancer patients died following thoraco-scopic pleurodesis as a result of their basic condition. In one of these patients, in addition to talc pleurodesis, a lung parenchyma fistula caused by a tumour had been successfully closed 18 days earlier.

– One patient who had undergone pneu-monectomy owing to a necrotizing bronchial carcinoma died of acute respiratory distress syndrome (ARDS). A barotrauma due to ven-tilation led to contralateral pneumothorax with extensive bullous changes of the com-plete remaining lobe; this could not be closed thoracoscopically since it was impossible to induce an adequate pneumothorax.

– In one patient who died of acute dissecting aneurysm of the aorta 2 days after thoraco-scopy, the autopsy revealed no injury to the aorta or to the parietal pleura covering it caused by thoracoscopic instruments. A com-plication arising from gas insufflation could also be ruled out since the routine chest X-rays taken 24 h after the operation showed no mediastinal emphysema and no dilation of the aorta with the lungs expanded.

The exact breakdown of our complications (Table 6) shows that the majority of clinically relevant complications were of a technical nature, and they can be avoided with more experience. Most complications involved bleeding with resulting haemothorax and injuries to the lung parenchyma caused by the introduction of the first trocar. Trocar injuries to the lung did not, however, lead to any significant bleeding, in all three cases of bleeding this resulted from injured intercostal ves-sels (Fig. 19).

Circumscribed subcutaneous emphysema is seen particularly following operations performed

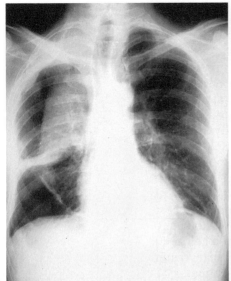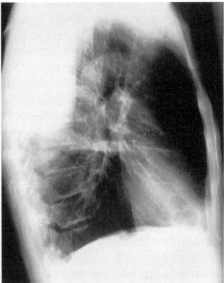

a   b

Fig. 19. a,b Dorsoapical
haemothorax extending
into the transverse fissure
following thoracoscopic
pleurectomy.
a Posteroanterior view.
b Lateral view

under local anaesthesia and is caused by fits of
coughing triggered by the vagus nerve forcing air
or gas into thoracic incisions. This is not uncommon, but nevertheless harmless. The only generalized air emphysema in our series developed
postoperatively. The massive expansion involving the mediastinum could only be relieved by a
transcervical mediastinotomy and multiple subcutaneous drainage. The drain placed in the encapsulated bed of the effusion in this cancer patient
never transported air despite the rapid progres-
sion of the emphysema. The probable explanation
is that as a trocar was inserted concave, atelectatic
lung parenchyma adhering to the thoracic wall
had been penetrated. The resulting leak must
have led to a loss of air along the inner thoracic
wall in a mediastinal direction and subcutaneously
through the incision.

In one patient, a tension pneumothorax developed 14 days after extensive resection of bullous pulmonary tissue. This had to be treated as
an emergency by means of a chest drain.

In one case of a spontaneous pneumothorax
with total collapse of the lung, which was neg-

lected by the patient for over a month, the thoracoscopic evacuation of the pneumothorax and
expansion of the completely conglutinated lung
led to a clinically irrelevant but nevertheless radiologically clearly visible interstitial pulmonary
oedema in the right middle lobe. In one female
patient, the fourth intercostal nerve was injured
during a thoracic sympathectomy causing unpleasant radicular hypaesthesia and dysaesthesia
in the affected area (cf. Chap. 14).

In one young patient with a spontaneous
pneumothorax and under local anaesthesia, the
lung was thoracoscopically unremarkable and 2 l
of Ringer's solution were instilled into the chest
cavity to aid the search for a leak. Without any
further manipulation a sinus bradycardia below 40
beats per minute and lasting more than 4 min
occurred, but was not noticed by the patient.

A harmless effect of thoracoscopy in many
patients is a febrile temperature without clinical
correlate in the first 48 h [20, 23, 70]. This affected
21% of our patients. The search for a local wound
infection or postthoracoscopic pleural empyema
did not produce any findings.

5 Prevention of Thrombosis and Prophylactic Antibiotics

5.1 Prevention of Thrombosis

If there are no special risks or indications involved, we base our measures for preventing thrombosis on those of open thoracic surgery in patients undergoing thoracoscopy under general anaesthesia. These patients are given s.c. low-molecular heparin perioperatively. Preoperatively the patients are instructed to perform physiotherapeutic exercises to flex and extend the calf muscles and to systematically exercise their lower extremities. Postoperative mobilization begins on the day of the operation. When we perform thoracoscopies under local anaesthesia, we do not give any special prophylactics. Up to now we have seen no clinically manifest deep vein thrombosis. We have also had no case of clinically detectable pulmonary embolism.

5.2 Prophylactic Antibiotics

Thirty-five patients were being treated with antibiotics for various reasons when referred for thoracoscopy.

We do not normally give antibiotics as a prophylactic measure, but have made exceptions to this in 28 cases up to now for patients undergoing immunotherapy, patients with disease of the immune system or those suffering from exacerbated chronic bronchitis and patients undergoing thoracoscopy for the resection of bullous tissue in cases of extensive pulmonary emphysema. These patients receive one single perioperative dose of a second-generation cephalosporin. To date, we have had neither postoperative infections in the area of the incisions nor infectious pleurisy or even empyema. One patient later reported that she had had a painful reddening of the skin in the area of the hemithorax operated on, although fever remained absent and she had been given antibiotics by her own GP.

6 Prerequisites for Performing Surgical Thoracoscopy

The patient, surgeon and hospital must meet a number of requirements before an operative thoracoscopy can be performed with acceptable risk factors.

Patient
With complete, histologically organized obliteration of the pleural cavity, thoracoscopy is impossible. Prior to performing operative thoracoscopy, global respiratory insufficiency, untreated, serious cardiac arrhythmias, recent myocardial infarction and clotting disorders with a prothrombin test value below 40% and a platelet count below $40\,000\,mm^3$ must be excluded. Before operating under general anaesthesia, the patient must be assessed "fit for anaesthesia". However, with care and experience, circumscribed diagnostic or therapeutic interventions are possible in patients considered unfit for intubation providing the patient will benefit from the operation (e.g. talc pleurodesis for treatment of malignant effusions).

Doctor
Doctors who intend to perform a thoracoscopy must have had suitable pneumological or surgical training. It is advisable to attend courses and seminars at which endoscopic techniques can be learned and practised. To sharpen diagnostic abilities, physicians interested in minimally invasive surgery can learn a lot from the wide experience of pneumologists who practise thoracoscopy. There is a wealth of literature on the subject, and excellent books and atlases are available [21, 26, 27, 169].

Infrastructure

While for diagnostic and interventional thoracoscopy it must be at least possible to call in surgeons
who can convert to open surgical methods, for
minimally invasive interventions these skills must
be immediately available. The infrastructure must
allow for fast conversion to an open surgical procedure at any time. The wards must also be
equipped with vacuum and oxygen connections.

7 Documentation – Methods and Uses

Thanks to electronic transmission and storage facilities, the possibilities of documenting endoscopic findings and operative procedures are almost unlimited. Video recorders allow the whole operation to be recorded on tape. If questions arise, the tape can be reviewed and evaluated. Various types of video printers can provide hard copies of the main pathological findings, interesting anatomical variations and specific steps in the operation. The postoperative information for the physicians involved and for the patient is both simplified and far more objective. Including this pictorial information in the operation report adds a new precision to the case history. Slides, photographs and tapes support and illustrate the spoken word in a teaching situation.

Table 7. Structure of the operation report

Diagnosis
Intervention performed
Anaesthetic technique used
Operating time
Indication for operation
Thoracosocopic technique used (description of technical procedure)

Thoracoscopic findings
  Amount of effusion and type
  Pleural space: free; adhesions; loculations
  Parietal pleura
  Mediastinum
  Diaphragm
  Recesses
  Lungs: lobes, fissures

Postoperative management

Dokumentation

Thorakoskopische Eingriffe

Der Arbeitsgemeinschaft für Laparo-
und Thorakoskopische Chirurgie

'92

Name (Blockschrift)	
Vorname	
Land / PLZ / Ort	
Strasse	Tel.
Beruf	Sprache
Versicherung	Behandelnder Arzt

Legende:
AB Antibiotika
BV Bildverstärker
COPD Chronisch obstruktive Pneumopathie
CT Computertomographie
DL Doppellumen-Tubus
FNP Feinnadelpunktion
HA Hausarzt
ICR Interkostalraum
LA Lokalanästhesie
LE Lungenembolie
Lufu Lungenfunktionsprüfung
Rx Röntgen
St. n. Status nach
TS Thorakoskopie
TU Tumor
TVT Tiefe Venenthrombose
US Ultraschall

Pneumothorax-Klassifikation n Vanderschueren:
I normale Lunge, keine Bullae, kein Leck sichtbar
II pleuro-pulmonale Adhäsionen
III kleine (<2 cm) Bullae vorhanden
IV grosse (>2 cm) Bullae, zahlreich

Patientenidentifikation: (rows 1–12, digits 0–9)

Geburtsdatum: Tag / Jan Feb Mär Apr Mai Jun Jul Aug Sep Okt Nov Dez / 18 19 20 '00 10 20 30 40 50 60 70 80 90

Geschl.: M W **Klinik-Nr./Belegarzt-Nr.:** 0–9

Praeoperative ASA-Risikogruppen
1 Normaler, sonst gesunder Patient
2 Patient mit leichter Systemerkrankung ohne Leistungseinschränkung
3 Patient mit schwerer Systemerkrankung mit Leistungseinschränkung
4 Patient mit schwerer Systemerkrankung, die mit oder ohne Operation das Leben des Patienten bedroht
5 Moribunder Patient, Tod innerhalb von 24 Stunden mit oder ohne Operation zu erwarten

Gewicht (kg) <40 48 58 69 79 89 99 109 119 129 >130
Grösse (cm) <150 155 160 165 170 175 180 185 190 195 200 >201
ASA Klassifikation 1 2 3 4 5

Eintrittsdatum: / **Datum des Haupteingriffs:** Tag Monat Jahr / **Entlassungsdatum:**

▼ Kommentar betreffend markierte Felder   Zusätzlicher Kommentar ▼

(1) Präoperativ

Eintritt	1 m [1]	Wahl- / Notfall- / Ambulant — 0 1
Indikation	1 + m [2]	Raumforderung: Thorax w. / Diaphragma / Lunge / Mediastinum — Lungenveränderung: umschrieben / diffus / unklar — Erguss: maligne / postaktinisch / anderer / Chylothorax
		Empyem / Hämato-thorax / Pneumothorax: rechts / links / 1. / Rezidivpneumothorax: 2. / 3. / >3 / persistierender Pneu — 0 2
Vorbest. Krankheiten	allg. 1 + m [3]	Hyperhidrose / Raynaud / Sudeck / Andere x — Nicotinabusus / Diabetes mellitus / Autoimmunerkrankung / metast. Malignom / Allergie x / andere x — 0 3
		keine / Hypertonie / Kardiopathie
	pulm. 1 + m [4]	keine / COPD / Aethma bronchiale: intr. / extr. / Pneumonie / Pleuritis / St. n. Thoraxtrauma / St.n. LE / St. n. pulm. Tumor / andere x — 0 4
Präop. Abklärung	1 + m [5]	keine / Rx Thorax / CT Thorax / Ultraschall: extern /)trans(/ transösophageal / skopie — Pleurapunktion / Pleuradrainage / St. n. Mediastinotomie / Me-diastinoskopie / andere x — 0 5
		FNP / Lavage / Zytologie: Bürste / Andere x / Lunge / Bronchien / Pleura / Lokalisation Zytologie: Mediastinum / präop. / andere x / Lufu

(2) Operation

Wahloperation/NF-Op Anästhesie	2 + m [6]	Wahl-Op / NF-Op / LA / Analgesie: intrapleural / i. v.-Sedation / Anästhesie stand-by / Endo-Intubation / DL-Intubation / andere x — 0 6
Anlage Pneumothorax	3 + m [7]	Pneu offen / Pneu geschlossen / Zimmer-Luft / Gas: CO_2 / anderes x / Endo-Insufflator / Hand-pumpe / Pneu-apparat / andere x — 0 7
Operateur Erfahrung	2 m [8]	Belegaz./ Chefaz. / Operateur: Leit. Az / Oberaz. / Ass. az / Gastaz. / TS-Erfahrung: <10 / 11–30 / 31–50 / 51–100 / >100 — 0 8
Op-Dauer Lage/BV Zugänge/Einblick	6 + m [9]	gesamte Op-Dauer: <30' / 31–60' / 61–90' / 91–120' / >120' x / Lage: Rücken- / Seiten- / Andere x / Bildverstärker: nein / intraop. / postop.
		Zugänge: 1 / 2 / 3 / 4 / >4 / Interkostalraum: 3. 4. 5. 6. 7. 8.
		ICR Anderer x / Einblick: vollständig / partiell / partieller Einblick wegen: Adhäsionen x / Obliteration / anderem x — 0 9

x erfordert Klartext

1.92 © AO-Dokumentationszentrale, CH-3000 Bern 14   Printed in Switzerland / BDB 26276

◄ **Fig. 20.** Documentation
form for thoracoscopy

Despite the pictorial documentation, the operation report remains the personal record of the operator. To make relevant information readily available, it is worth the effort to keep to a clear structure. We use the structure shown in Table 7.

The future position of minimally invasive methods in thoracic surgery is not yet decided. A listing of possible indications, studies of the operative techniques, compilations of all reported complications and evaluations of long-term results are imperative. Only then is fruitful discussion and comparison with traditional procedures possible, paving the way for an objective assessment.

With this goal in mind, we have designed a computer questionnaire which allows the collection and centralized evaluation of standardized and comprehensive patient data (Fig. 20). This project has been sponsored by the Swiss study group for laparoscopic and thoracoscopic surgery. The technical know-how for the undertaking was kindly provided by the Swiss study group for osteosynthesis (AO), a group that has been using such documentation successfully for many years to provide continuous quality control and further developments in the operative treatment of fractures.

B Specific Techniques

8 Thoracoscopy in Diagnosis

8.1 General

The possibility of exploring the thoracic cavity and its structures directly and of obtaining biopsies from specific areas, swabs and specimens of effusion followed up by histological, cytological, microbiological, immunological and chemical analysis, makes thoracoscopy a valuable addition to the diagnostic arsenal of the practising pneumologist [41, 115, 174]. The most common indications and the results obtained can be seen in Table 8. In addition to the diagnostic thoracoscopies listed, in six patients with histologically verified bronchial carcinoma, oncological staging included the thoracoscopic dissection of a suspicious aorto-pulmonary lymph node (N2) which was followed by a planned mini-thoracotomy to verify the thoracoscopic findings.

Table 8. Indications and results of diagnostic thoracoscopy

Indication	Patients (n)	Successful diagnosis (n)
Diffuse malignant mesothelioma	11	11/11
Tumour		
Pleural (malignant/benign: 13/8)	21	21/21
Mediastinal (malignant/benign: 3/5)	8	7/8[a]
Pulmonary findings		
Circumscribed (malignant/benign: 5/8)	13	9/13[b]
Diffuse (malignant/benign: 1/10)	11	11/11
Unexplained chronic effusion (malignant/benign: 2/6)	8	8/8

[a] Thoracotomy in the same anaesthesia owing to inconclusive frozen section (pericardial cyst)
[b] In two patients thoracotomy in the same anaesthesia owing to inconclusive frozen section (one old, scarred spherical atelectasis, subpleural and one old fibrous intraparenchymatous scar)

It is not possible at present to stipulate the position of thoracoscopy among the diagnostic methods. As a guideline one can say that it is indicated as a diagnostic tool whenever imaging techniques and fine-needle biopsy have not led to a conclusive diagnosis. The thoracoscopic instrument set available today allows biopsies of any size to be taken. It can therefore often replace an explorative or diagnostic thoracotomy. The complete view of the thoracic cavity afforded by endoscopy would only otherwise be possible with an extended thoracotomy.

8.2 Operative Procedure

The patient position, anaesthesia, induction of pneumothorax and establishment of the sites of entry are as described in the previous chapters. An adequate view of all intrathoracic structures is vital for an accurate diagnosis. Adhesions should therefore be divided with appropriate care. Only then can the search for pathological changes and suspicious structures begin.

Biopsy by Ligature (Fig. 21a). Peripherally located tumours and altered sections of the lung can be grasped by the parenchyma forceps, pulled

Fig. 21a,b. Lung biopsy with ligature (**a**), and with stapler (**b**)

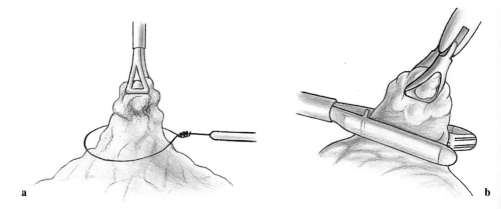

a   b

through a Roeder loop (chromic catgut) and divided from the lung parenchyma both airtight and without bleeding (Fig. 22 a–c). The specimen is cut with the scissors between 3 and 5 mm distal to the ligature. If the ligature is not clearly peripheral as for example in the lingula or in segment 5 of the left lower lobe, it should be covered with fast-acting fibrin glue (1 ml Tissucol). Care must be taken to ensure that the fibrin layer is kept thin, otherwise it will slip off when the lung is re-expanded, if not before [152].

If malignancy is suspected, the biopsy must be evacuated in a plastic bag (Fig. 23). Specimens of atelectatic lung tissue up to a diameter of approximately 2.5 cm can be extracted easily through the mini-incision after removing the trocar sleeve. The intercostal musculature is forced apart and the skin is sufficiently elastic to expand. For larger biopsies, the intercostal musculature can be expanded slightly with the scissors and the skin incision extended to 2–2.5 cm.

Biopsy with the Stapler (Fig. 21b). If larger-area parenchymal biopsies are required, the less expensive ligature must be replaced by the Endo-GIA stapler (Autosuture). The technique of wedge resection is described in Chap. 9. The methods of removing the specimen are the same as those described above.

Biopsy by Sharp Excision. If the pulmonary pathology is such that it is technically impossible or difficult to obtain a biopsy by ligature or wedge resection, the selected tissue can be raised with the parenchyma forceps and then cut out using scissors. Care must be taken not to cut too deep into the parenchyma to avoid injury to larger pulmonary vessels. For the same reason, biopsies in the fissure areas are also dangerous. To prevent a persistent pulmonary leak or bleeding, we carefully inject 1–2 ml fast-acting fibrin glue below the excised area (Fig. 24). The reusable cannula must be thoroughly rinsed with Ringer's solution immediately after use to avoid an irreversible reduction of the lumen by dried fibrin glue.

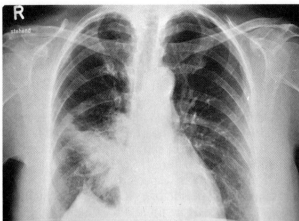

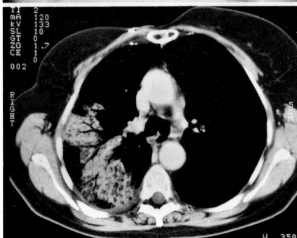

Fig. 22. a Radiograph of the thorax: atelectatic middle lobe and pulmonary infiltration of unclear aetiology. **b** CT scan. **c** Endoscopic image: part of the atelectatic middle lobe ligated and prepared for biopsy. **d, e** Taking the biopsy from the middle lobe. The histological diagnosis was a scirrhous adenocarcinoma of the breast which had caused a chronic interstitial and alveolar pneumonia. Repeated fine-needle biopsies had failed to produce conclusive results

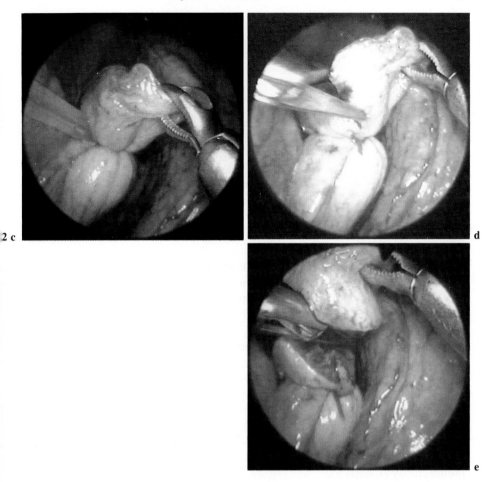

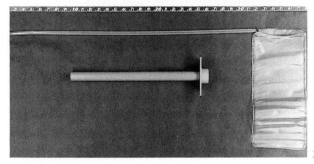

Fig. 23. Plastic bag for removing resected specimens (Ethicon)

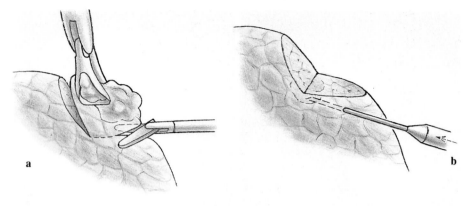

Each biopsy is completed by irrigating the site and checking for complete haemostasis. Surface bleeding is coagulated with the mini grasping forceps.

Fig. 24. a Lung biopsy with scissors. **b** Sealing the surface of the lung by injecting the parenchyma with fibrin glue (fast-acting components)

Pleural Biopsy. These can be grasped as circumscribed multiple biopsies with the monopolar biopsy forceps and then coagulated using the technique described by Boutin et al. [21] or they are incised with the coagulation probe and dissected in the avascular layer on the endothoracic fascia with the dissector and then resected. The surgical technique corresponds to that used for parietal pleurectomy (Chap. 9).

Intrathoracic Tumours and Cysts (see Chap. 15)

Mediastinal Biopsies. If the findings are clearly circumscribed and superficial, the covering of mediastinal pleura is first opened with the coagulation probe. Depending on the consistency of the tissue, the scissors, dissector (disintegrated tissue) or a grasping forceps are used to take sufficient material as far as possible without compressing it. Haemostasis is achieved by specific coagulation with the mini forceps. By simultaneously irrigating the biopsy site, diffuse bleeding such as encountered with lymphomas can also be stopped.

Up to now we have exposed mediastinal lymph nodes in the aorto-pulmonary window in the course of tumour staging (TNM) in five patients to clarify N2 involvement. The endoscopic intervention was followed by a planned parasternal thoracotomy to verify the endoscopic dissection and to take the required biopsies. We are currently evaluating endoscopic mediastinal lymph node dissection as a staging method analogous to mediastinoscopy.

Diagnostic thoracoscopy is completed in the usual manner. After taking biopsies, drains with a diameter less than 24 Fr. should not be used since blood clots and exudate could otherwise block them.

8.3 Our Own Experience

Up to now we have taken larger biopsies 72 times either as the sole manoeuvre or in conjunction with therapeutic measures. Twice the thoracoscopy had to be abandoned owing to obliteration of the pleural cavity (2.94%). In three patients (including those with obliteration) no diagnosis was possible and in three further cases frozen sections failed to produce conclusive evidence with regard to malignancy (8.82%). In these cases we converted to thoracotomy which permitted a diagnosis in each case.

Thoracoscopy was used seven times to exclude a T4 staging as defined in the TNM system. The purpose of the interventions was to search for pleural tumour spreading or to obtain a diagnosis of suspicious intrapulmonary findings which were not accessible to fine-needle puncture (cf. Chap. 15). In approximately 20%–25% of patients with bronchial carcinoma, a reliable diagnosis is often impossible without an open biopsy via a thoracotomy despite the variety of existing diagnostic methods (e.g. transbronchial, percutaneous needle biopsy) [157]. Thoracoscopy can be used in such cases as a less invasive method. The case of a female patient with indurated pulmonary metastases from a carcinoma of the breast which had been operated on 3 years previously illustrates this point. The metastases could not be detected bronchoscopically nor by fine-needle biopsy (Fig. 22a–c).

In the 64 patients who underwent thoracoscopy exclusively for diagnostic purposes, the drain was usually removed on the first postoperative day. The average drainage time was 40 h (0–130 h). Analysis of the postoperative hospitalization times is meaningless, since many of these patients underwent thoracoscopy within the course of comprehensive diagnostic evaluation and remained in hospital for quite some time afterwards.

8.4 Possible Complications

Chapter 4 deals with the complications of operative thoracoscopy. In our series of diagnostic interventions we only encountered one complication. A 35-year-old patient with persistent pleuritic pain and a radiologically demonstrable right-sided basal pulmonary shadow, which on thoracoscopy proved to be an older pulmonary infarction in the process of organizing, developed a haemothorax which was evacuated via a minithoracotomy under local anaesthesia.

8.5 Other Thoracoscopic Methods

Apart from the technique using rigid thoracoscopes via one port (with an operating thoracoscope) or two ports, which have been established for decades by schools of pneumological thoracoscopy [11, 21, 23, 25, 150, 161, 162], methods have also been developed, particularly by surgeons, using a mediastinoscope [39, 101, 110, 123, 183]. In addition, video thoracoscopy has now found its place in diagnostic thoracoscopy among the pneumologists as well [21].

As discussed above, thoracoscopic techniques are also suitable for preoperative oncological assessment in cases of bronchial carcinoma when the relationship of the primary tumour to its surroundings is unclear despite imaging techniques, when there is cytologically undefined accompanying effusion with suspected pleural spread or when no conclusive diagnosis can be made. Since Brandt and Loddenkemper pointed out these possibilities, reports of the use of such methods have become increasingly common [7, 14, 22, 26, 31–33, 50, 109, 156, 176, 186]. The use of video techniques with the possibility of uncomplicated documentation also fulfils a useful function.

Boutin et al. [21] deal with the thoracoscopic diagnosis of mesothelioma and endoscopic therapeutic concepts in great detail.

9 Spontaneous Pneumothorax

9.1 General

Pneumothorax is defined as the entry of air into the pleural cavity due to a leak in the visceral or parietal pleura. In spontaneous pneumothorax there is a discontinuity of the visceral pleural membrane. It is termed idiopathic or primary when it occurs without any clinically recognizable cause. Several theories have been put forward regarding its aetiology, including elastic fibre defects of the supporting tissue [8] or a discrepancy between the growth rate of the lung parenchyma and that of the vascular system [187]. The condition particularly affects young men. Physical exertion as the cause of the tear in the visceral pleura has never been conclusively proved. Of the 178 patients we treated between 1980 and 1990, extreme physical activity could only be considered a possible factor in 5%. In its symptomatic (secondary) form, pneumothorax is the result of a variety of pulmonary diseases such as chronic obstructive pneumopathy, bronchial asthma, bronchiectasis, or mucoviscidosis.

The generally accepted strategy for treating the first episode is simple drainage. If the condition persists, either chemical pleurodesis is induced by introducing various agents (such as tetracycline [120], talc [64], or fibrin [73]) via the indwelling drain or thoracoscopically, or operative therapy is recommended [40, 56, 57]. The classical surgical treatment of complicated (persisting or recurrent) spontaneous pneumothorax with extensive parenchymal alteration is resection of the leak or bulla in conjunction with parietal pleurectomy [28, 40]. As promising alternatives, resection of isolated open bullae [102] or of bullae up to 2 cm in diameter, thoracoscopic treatment of

Fig. 25. Algorithm for treatment of spontaneous pneumothorax (*DL*, double-lumen)

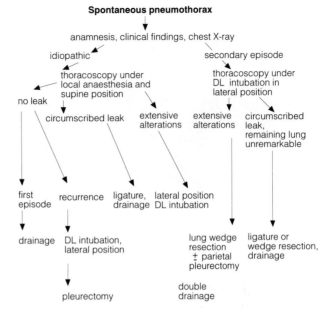

the bullae by coagulation [177] and talc dusting [64] have been described.

Minimally invasive operating techniques allow complete thoracoscopic treatment of spontaneous pneumothorax. We determine the thoracoscopic procedure at the first clinical evaluation according to the algorithm shown in Fig. 25.

9.2 Operative Procedure

Bulla Ligature [81, 82, 84] (Fig. 26). If the patient's medical history, the clinical findings and the chest radiograph strongly suggest an idiopathic spontaneous pneumothorax, we begin the intervention with the patient in the supine position under local anaesthesia. Prior to the intervention, patients are informed about their condition and the intended operation and their consent is obtained to induce a general anaesthesia and extend the scope of the thoracoscopy as necessary. The

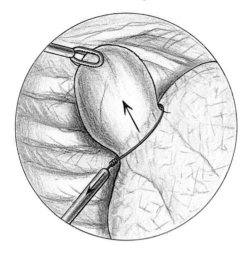

Fig. 26. Ligature of a bulla with a Roeder loop (chromic catgut)

patient must also be informed of the possibility of a thoracotomy if unexpected complications occur.

Supine Position, Local Infiltration Anaesthesia With or Without I.V. Sedation, Three Standard Sites of Entry. After dividing any adhesions, the first step is the general thoracoscopic examination of the structures. Pathological changes are usually found in the apical and apicodorsal areas and less often at the upper margin of the middle and inferior lobes. In idiopathic spontaneous pneumothorax, other locations are extremely rare. Circumscribed small blebs or bullae are grasped and their bases ligated with a chromic catgut Roeder loop, leaving an adequate margin of healthy parenchyma. If the lesion is clearly limited and does not exceed approximately 4 cm in diameter, our experience up to now has shown that the less expensive Roeder loop can safely be used rather than the stapler. Multiple blebs and bullae with adequate space between them can be treated in this way.

If a leak is found, the patient should be asked to cough. Collapsed blebs or blisters usually turn out to be leaks. If this produces no result, the "water test" may help in some cases (cf. Sect. 3.10). A promising technique is the leak test with preoperative inhalation of fluorescein as described by Boutin et al. [17]. After applying a simple leak ligature it is sufficient to insert a chest drain through the most caudal incision at the end of the intervention (cf. Fig. 13). This allows complete evacuation of the air after the leak has been sealed. After careful expansion of the lung under vision, all the trocar sleeves are removed and the other two incisions closed by single knotted sutures. The sterile conditions at the operating table are maintained until the drainage system is functioning (cf. Sect. 3.7). When this is correctly installed no further air should escape through the water seal after the lung has re-expanded. If this is not the case, it is advisable to have a second look at the lung endoscopically.

Wedge Resection [83, 84] (Fig. 27). If extensive changes are found on thoracoscopy under local anaesthesia for which simple ligatures would be unsatisfactory or which cannot be clearly differentiated from the surrounding healthy parenchyma, a wedge resection of the affected sections of lung is performed.

Lateral Position, Double-Lumen Intubation. The standard entry sites are usually topographically suitable. If bullous changes were located radiologically or by computed tomography scan in the basal sections of the lung in preparation for an

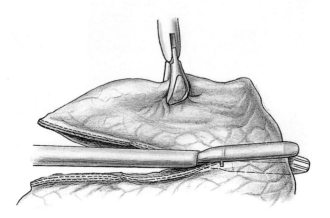

Fig. 27. Wedge resection of the lung with the stapler

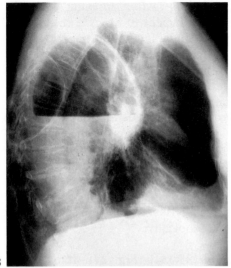

28

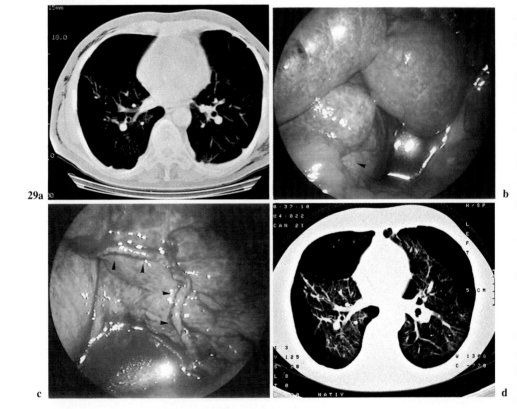

29a

b

c

d

◀ **Fig. 28.** Lateral view
radiograph of a patient
with persistent secondary
(pulmonary emphysema)
pneumothorax with
infected bullae following
long-term drainage

Fig. 29. a Preoperative
CT scan of pulmonary
emphysema with fibrosis
of the lung.
b Intraoperative findings:
view of the base of the left
lung. Beside the bullae,
mediastinal fat (*yellow/
orange*) can be seen
(*arrow*) from the area of
the phrenicomediastinal
recess. **c** Intraoperative
finding after
thoracoscopic bulla
resection. The rows of
staples (*arrows*) were
additionally sealed with
fibrin glue. **d** Ten days
after the operation: CT
scan at the same level.
Left, the remaining
parenchyma has spread
after resection of bullous
parts of the lung

elective intervention, as can occur in a secondary
pneumothorax resulting from emphysematous
bullae, the sites of one or two of the incisions are
selected in lower intercostal spaces or extra sites
established to gain unobstructed access to this
region. Figure 28 shows the preoperative X-ray of
such a case. Figure 29 shows the situation before
and after resection of bullous lung sections in the
left basal region of the lung.

If, following the exploration, we decide to
perform a wedge resection, one of the 7 mm trocar
sleeves is replaced by the special 12 mm sleeve
belonging to the stapler. To avoid possible injury
to the lung and mediastinal structures with the
larger calibre sharp-tipped trocar, it must be introduced extremely carefully and under strict endoscopic control. The Endo-GIA 30 is then inserted
and opened. The section of lung to be resected
is carefully placed between the branches of the
stapler with the parenchyma grasping forceps.
The line of resection must be in healthy paren-
chymatous tissue to ensure that the suture is as
airtight as possible. Before closing the stapler, the
parenchyma should lie loosely in the head of
the instrument. After the combined firing/cutting
manoeuvre, the Endo-GIA is cautiously closed
before it is removed to avoid unnecessary loss
of metal staples. The instrument can be used
for further resections by loading new magazines
(blue). Parts of the visceral pleura not completely
divided are carefully cut with scissors as far as the
last clip. The resected tissue is then removed
through the 12 mm incision using the parenchyma
grasping forceps.

The airtightness of the suture can be checked
using the water test. If a larger leak is found, an
additional staple suture is advisable. Smaller leaks
can be closed with fast-acting fibrin glue after
aspirating the fluid (cf. Chap. 2). The intervention
is completed as usual by placing a closed air drain
ventroapically.

Parietal Pleurectomy [84, 85]. If no leak can be
found in a recurrent or persistent pneumothorax,
if there are extensive bullous changes or bullae

difficult to differentiate from surrounding healthy tissue or if the pneumothorax is associated with generalized pulmonary disease, e.g. mucoviscidosis, a parietal pleurectomy is indicated.

Lateral Position, Double-Lumen Intubation, Three Standard Entry Sites. After the exploration of the thoracic cavity and ligature or resection of bullae to seal any leaks, the lines of resection are defined for the intended pleurectomy (Fig. 30a). The boundaries of the resection depend on the extent of the altered lung sections. Normally, this involves the apical parts of the upper lobe and less often the upper margin of the middle and/or lower lobe. The fifth rib is therefore usually adequate as the caudal limit for a satisfactory pleurectomy. The basal lung sections vital for ventilation then remain unaffected. The longitudinal limit of the resection runs in the apical direction along the sympathetic trunk as far as the height of the left subclavian artery or the brachiocephalic trunk on the right. To avoid thermal damage to the sympathetic trunk caused by the coagulation probe, a lateral clearance of 1 cm is maintained for the pleural incision (Fig. 30b). The pleura is grasped with the parenchyma grasping forceps (or with the mini grasping forceps if the pleura is delicate), raised and divided with a dissector in the avascular layer on the endothoracic fascia (Fig. 30c). A T-shaped incision at the height of the large vessels (Fig. 30d) allows controlled wing-like dissection in the area of the inlet of the thorax without damaging neighbouring vessels and nerves.

The pleural membrane can then be removed easily through the trocar sleeve in three pieces. As routine, these should be sent for histology. After thorough haemostasis and checking that there are no large leaks in the parenchyma, an air and fluid drain (24 and 28 Fr.) are placed through the existing incisions. To achieve optimal placement of the dorsobasal fluid drain we use curved tubes (Fig. 13). The intervention is completed in the usual manner.

Fig. 30. **a** Extension of the thoracoscopic parietal pleurectomy and adjacent anatomical structures. **b** Incision of the pleura with the coagulation hook. *Yellow*, sympathetic trunk. **c** Removing the pleura from the endothoracic fascia. **d** T-shaped incision in the pleura at the height of the subclavian artery or brachiocephalic trunk allows wing-like dissection in the area of the thoracic inlet

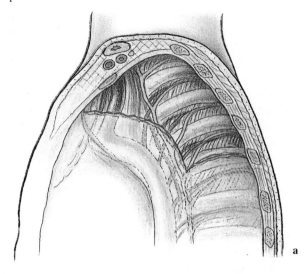

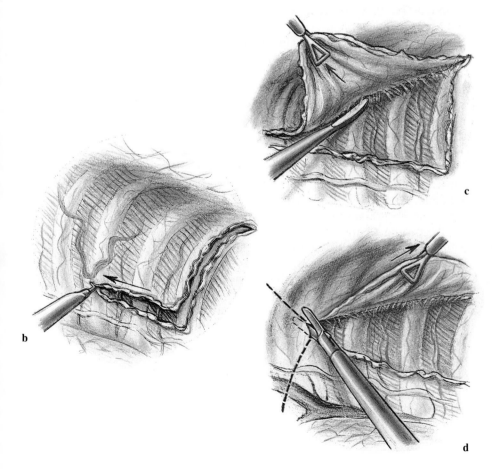

9.3 Our Own Experience

Since January 1990 we have performed thoracoscopy for spontaneous pneumothorax in 78 patients. In the first 16 patients, we restricted the
intervention to gaining an endoscopic overview
followed by fibrin or talc pleurodesis. If extensive
bullous changes were discovered, the bullae were
resected in the same session by means of a transaxillary mini-thoracotomy. As it became possible
to apply an endoscopic ligature (a strong chromic
catgut loop and a step-by-step ligature technique
are essential for large bullae) and to perform
endoscopic parietal pleurectomy, from March
1990 onwards all patients were treated exclusively
by thoracoscopy according to the algorithm described above. From July 1991, the use of staplers
extended the thoracoscopic technique to include
wedge resection.

To date we have treated 62 patients in this
way (18 women and 44 men) ranging in age from
16 to 81 years (average 36 years). In 23 cases,
the pneumothorax episode was clearly caused
by pulmonary disease, including two cases of
mucoviscidosis, while 39 cases were classified as
idiopathic. The average monitoring time is currently 10.6 months (1–27 months) covering the 2-
year period from March 1990 to 1992. Table 9
illustrates the thoracoscopic technique used, the
drainage times, postoperative hospitalization
times and any relapses and complications.

According to the algorithm (Fig. 25), young
patients with a first episode or patients referred to
us with persistent pneumothorax were operated
on 15 times under local anaesthesia and 10 times
under general anaesthesia at the patient's request.
Eight of the 25 patients were treated as day cases,
nine patients were hospitalized for longer than
24 h at their own request and a further eight were
kept in for observation owing to pain or high
temperature. In 22 of the 25 patients treated by
ligature, the drainage system could be removed
during the first postoperative day. Three required
drainage for between 96 and 120 h. Following
wedge resection one female patient required a

Table 9. Pneumothorax: thoracosocopic technique in 62 patients

Thoracoscopic technique	Number of patients (n)	Operating time (min)		Drainage time (h)		Postoperative hospitalization		Relapses (n)
		Range	Mean	Range	Mean	Range	Mean	
Overview	3	20–40	28	24–72	40	1–9	5.3	–
Ligature	25	15–70	36	0–120	30	Day–6	2.2	2
Wedge resection	12	30–60	38	1–240	41	1–9	4.1	–
Pleurectomy	22	45–90	56	24–72	47	2–13	3.9	1

Day, outpatient treatment

thorax drain for 9 days owing to a persistent air fistula. This was the only patient requiring drainage for longer than 48 h.

None of the complications resulting from thoracoscopy made a surgical intervention necessary. In two cases, postoperative radiological examinations revealed basal dystelectasis without clinical symptoms. One air leak persisted in the region of a staple suture. A haematoma in the oblique fissure, originating from highly vascularized apicodorsal adhesions, was reabsorbed within 4 weeks without further measures being necessary. These adhesions had been divided prior to pleurectomy. To locate a leak in a 17-year-old patient, 2 l of Ringer's solution were instilled under local anaesthesia without having been prewarmed. This led to an alarming vasovagal bradycardia below 40 beats per minute with the sinus rhythm retained. The rhythm recovered after 4 min without requiring intervention.

Three patients (4.8%) underwent a second thoracoscopy 5, 14 and 16 days, respectively after the first intervention to treat a recurrent pneumothorax. In two of these cases, no visible bulla had been located during the thoracoscopy under local anaesthesia. However, a circumscribed fibrin deposit which could not be stripped away had been discovered in the apical area and ligated along with the underlying lung tissue as a suspected leak. The third patient had returned to work as a self-employed driving instructor 3 days after a successful pleurectomy. The drains had

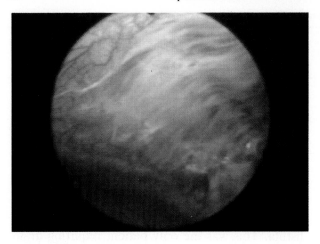

Fig. 31. Scarring of the endothoracic fascia resembling mother of pearl 7 days after pleurectomy in an early recurrence. The edges of the pleurectomy are clearly visible

been removed 24 h after the operation after radiology had confirmed an expanded lung and an effusion-free thoracic cavity. On the fifth day, the radiological check-up made by the patient's GP showed an encapsulated latero-apical pneumothorax. During the subsequent second thoracoscopy no overlooked bullae could be found. The pleurectomized thoracic wall in the area of the renewed circumscribed pneumothorax had already formed scar tissue which shone like mother of pearl (Fig. 31). On the basis of these findings we assume that if unrestricted physical activity is resumed too early, the trocar sites in the thin thoracic wall used as drainage ports and created without using a "Z" technique can allow air through and cause a circumscribed recurrence.

9.4 Conclusions

In the 62 patients treated thoracoscopically, the mean hospitalization time was 3.3 days, complication rates in the intra- and postoperative phases were low, and the early recurrence rate was 4.8%. In the overall statistics based on the literature, first episode spontaneous pneumothorax treated exclusively by drainage has a recurrence rate of 21% and simple observation in hospital a rate of

29% [21]. Over 70% of recurrences occur during the first 2 years [21, 60]. Although long-term results are not yet available to allow a definitive assessment of the method, in view of the good results achieved up to now, we nevertheless feel justified in evaluating all spontaneous pneumothoraces thoracoscopically.

The indications for this procedure in patients with idiopathic processes corresponding to Vanderschueren's stage I (Table 10, Fig. 32a–c), where no pathological changes in the lung can be detected thoracoscopically, remain inexact. In our series, this involved five patients (Table 11) and in the meantime two of our three recurrences belong to this group. In keeping with the remarks made by Boutin et al. [21], that during an exact examination of the so-called normal lung and careful endoscopic investigation of idiopathic pneumothoraces (Vanderschueren's stage I) it is often possible to recognize minute blebs and bullae, we have come to the conclusion that when thoracoscopic pathology is "absent", parietal pleurectomy with the informed preoperative consent of

Table 10. Thoracosopic staging of pneumothorax by Vanderschueren

Stage I	Stage II	Stage III	Stage IV
Idiopathic pneumothorax, endoscopically normal lung	Pneumothorax with pleuropulmonary adhesions	Pneumothorax with blebs and bullae, <2 cm diameter	Pneumothorax with numerous bullae >2 cm diameter

Table 11. Pneumothorax: aetiology and morphology

	Primary spontaneous pneumothorax				Secondary spontaneous pneumothorax			
Stages according to Vanderschueren	V1	V2	V3	V4	V1	V2	V3	V4
First episode (<7 days)	4	1	5	2	1	–	–	1
Persistent (>7 days)	–	–	6	3	–	2	1	6
Recurrent pneumothorax	–	2	6	10	–	1	1	10

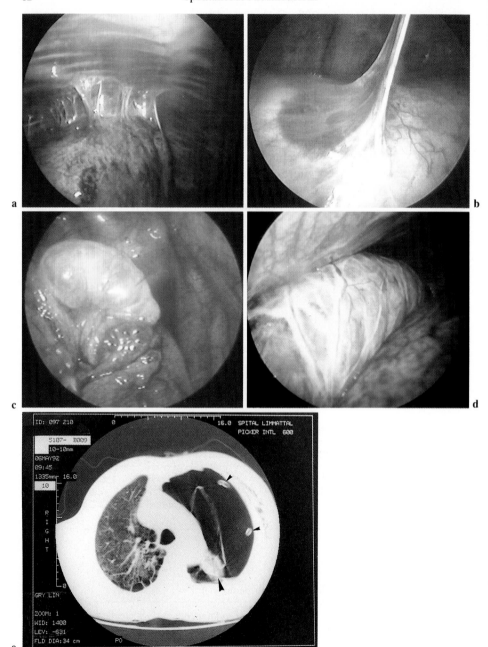

the patient is justified. If the patient requests it, we also terminate the intervention simply by placing a drain. This accounts for the three diagnostic thoracoscopies in our series. Boutin's fluorescein inhalation test may prove to be an additional aid in locating leaks. This involves the patient inhaling 10 ml of 20% fluorescein solution (NaCl 0.9%) from an aerosol 20 min before the thoracoscopy, so that leaks in the visceral pleura can be recognized as yellowish patches [17].

A total of 48 of the 62 patients were referred to our department with recurrent or persistent pneumothoraces lasting longer than 7 days. An acute first episode had been diagnosed in only 14 cases (cf. Table 11). Among these patients, three previous contralateral spontaneous pneumothoraces were known; serious pulmonary conditions (mucoviscidosis, pneumocystis carinii pneumonia) weighed heavily in the medical history of two patients, and we diagnosed one tension pneumothorax.

9.5 Other Thoracoscopic Methods

In the thoracoscopy literature, various techniques for treating pneumothorax have been reported. These include pleurodesis with fibrin [45, 73, 76, 94] and talc [21, 43, 64, 167], the latter achieving impressive results with a recurrence rate below 8% while the rate following fibrin treatment is quoted between 9% and 25%. Lasers are also finding increasing application in the therapy of spontaneous pneumothorax, both for sealing leaks in the lung and for combined treatment of the leak followed by pleural scarification [164].

Evaluation of the various techniques used is difficult owing to the different patient selection criteria and descriptions of the intraoperative findings, as well as the differences in the duration of postoperative drainage. Patients with lesions corresponding to Vanderschueren's stage IV are treated surgically in most of these series.

10 Haemothorax

10.1 General

In cases of haemothorax, the therapeutic procedure depends primarily on the cause and extent of the source of bleeding. If the intrathoracic haemorrhage is accumulating slowly and is not threatening the cardiovascular situation, a drain is normally placed both for therapy and to check the blood loss. Explorative thoracotomy is indicated if there is persistent blood loss greater than 500 ml/h for more than 3 h or 150 ml/h for 6 h through the chest tube [58]. If a haemothorax cannot be evacuated by drainage within a few days, operative evacuation is also necessary.

The search for a persistent source of bleeding and the evacuation of an old, often loculated haemothorax are indications for thoracoscopy (Figs. 33a,b, 34).

10.2 Operative Procedure

Pleural sensitivity to pain is generally greatly reduced by adherent blood clots, so that the intervention can often be performed under local anaesthesia. To be able to explore the phrenicocostal sinus safely and to free it of blood clots, a slightly raised lateral position under local anaesthesia is useful.

If the intervention is performed under general anaesthesia the patient is routinely placed in the lateral position. The three incisions are planned on the basis of posteroanterior and lateral view thoracic X-rays according to the position and extent of the haematoma.

Initially, approximately 300 ml CO_2 are carefully insufflated through the Verres needle. If the

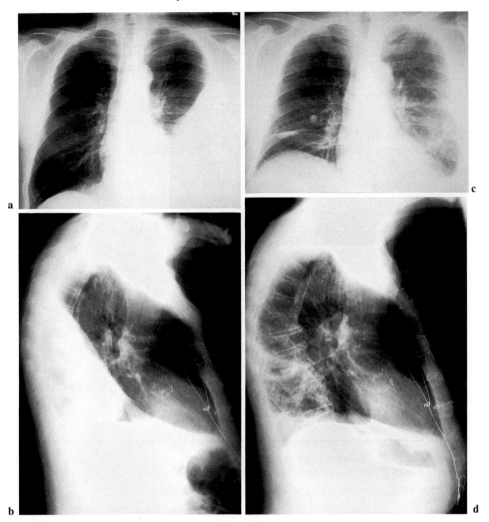

Fig. 33a–d. Haematoma after aortocoronary bypass operation.
a Thorax in posteroanterior view prior to thoracoscopy.
b Thorax in lateral view prior to thoracoscopy.
c After thoracoscopic evacuation, posteroanterior view.
d After thoracoscopic evacuation, lateral view

insufflation pressure is above 10 mmHg and/or gas flow is slow, blind gas insufflation is stopped since the tip of the cannula may be located in clotted blood. Instead an incision is made with the scissors and a trocar inserted to allow viewing with the 0° telescope. If the light is absorbed by the haematoma, parts of it are evacuated by alternate irrigation and suction. This quickly improves the lighting conditions. The next step is to define the anatomical structures and the boundaries of

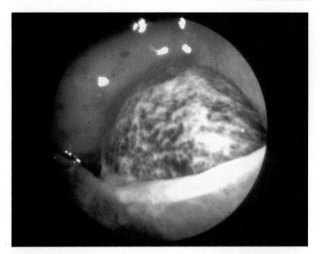

Fig. 34. Endoscopic image of an older encapsulated haematoma with a clearly visible pseudocapsule of fibrin

the haematoma to avoid further damage to lacerated lung parenchyma. Older haematomas often have membranes with a matt sheen resembling the visceral pleura of atelectatic regions of the lung (compare Fig. 34 and Fig. 22c).

If a source of bleeding is found (intercostal vessel, small vein) it is closed, if possible, with fibrin glue, a suture or clip. Before completion of the intervention it is important to make sure that the pulmonary fissures and recesses have been exposed and examined. They are often the site of encapsulated remnants of the haematoma.

10.3 Our Own Experience

Our material is represented in Table 12. With the exception of patients 3 and 6, all patients were treated with a thorax drain (32 Fr.) prior to thoracoscopy. Patient 8 underwent thoracoscopy owing to persistent bleeding and the others because satisfactory drainage was not achieved.

Table 12. Thoracoscopic treatment of haemothorax ($n = 8$)

Patient	Age (years)	Diagnosis	Time of thoracoscopy (days after event)	Thoracoscopic findings	Technique	Remarks
Male	26	Gunshot wound	5	Lacerations of lung, fibrin deposits	A,L,E,D	Pneumocele in postoperative X-ray
Male	59	Multiple rib fractures	5	Atelectasis of inferior lobe	A,L,E,D	Postoperative atelectasis expanded
Male	33	Iatrogenic after resection of first rib	17	Organized haematoma overlooked in thoracoscopy	A	Postoperative persistent atelectasis, fever, open decortication
Male	31	Multiple rib fractures	7	Lacerations of lung	A,L,E,D	
Female	57	Gunshot wound	10	Organized haematoma with capsule	A,L,E,D	
Male	84	Iatrogenic after AC bypass	10	Organized haematoma with capsule	A,L,E,D	cf. Fig. 31
Male	71	Dissecting aneurysm of aorta	7	Organized haematoma with capsule	A,L,E,D	
Male	59	Haemorrhage from intercostal artery after thoracoscopy	1	Bleeding from second intercostal artery, fresh haematoma	Coagulation, L,E,D	

A, adhesiolysis; L, lavage; E, evacuation; D, drain placed under vision; AC bypass, aortocoronary bypass

10.4 Conclusions

A haemothorax which cannot be adequately evacuated by drainage is a straightforward and safe indication for thoracoscopy. The extent and position of the haematoma can be determined easily by conventional radiology allowing advance planning of the intervention. The operator should also be on the lookout for other pathological findings such as atelectatic lung tissue (cf. patients 3 and 4) or lacerations of the lung parenchyma (cf. patients 1, 4, and 5). Anatomical landmarks such as the fissures must be examined to avoid overlooking atelectatic lung tissue trapped in the haematoma. If original sources of bleeding are located haemostasis can be attempted (cf. patient 8). If any doubt remains conversion to an open procedure should not be considered a "failure".

The decision to perform thoracoscopy should not be delayed too long since increasing organization makes the whole procedure more difficult (patient 3) and increases the hospitalization time unnecessarily.

10.5 Other Thoracoscopic Methods

Various authors describe thoracoscopic haemostasis using flexible endoscopes [42, 138]. Kaiser reports on thoracoscopic evacuation of haematomas using a mediastinoscope [893]. Both he and Jones et al. [92], who performed thoracoscopy to locate bleeding and evacuate clots in 32 patients as an emergency measure in traumatic haemothorax, point out the advantages of an early intervention. The absence of organization of the haematoma with little fibrin deposit allows complete evacuation and effective drainage of the thoracic cavity.

If thoracoscopy is performed according to the principles of minimally invasive surgery, the experience gained with lasers, which allow accurate haemostasis in the area of the lung parenchyma, represents an interesting prospect [107]. While closing bleeding pulmonary vessels, the air fistulae resulting from the lacerations can also be sealed. This, therefore, creates the conditions required for complete re-expansion of the lung and establishment of the physiological negative pressure in the pleural cavity.

11 Chylothorax

11.1 General

Postoperative chylothorax resulting from injury to the thoracic duct (Fig. 35a) is a relatively rare, but nevertheless well-known problem following oper-

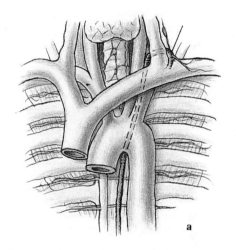

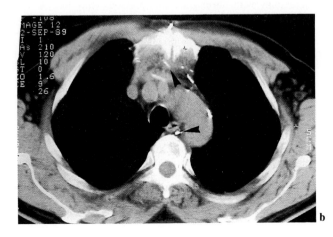

Fig. 35. a Intrathoracic route of the thoracic duct **b** Lymphangio-CT scan at the height of the outflow of contrast. *Arrows*, thoracic duct prevertebral and outflow of contrast

ations on the aorta, heart, lungs and oesophagus. The best therapeutic procedure for this situation is a matter of controversy. Conservative methods usually involve drainage and parenteral feeding. Despite substitution there is nevertheless a loss of proteins, fat-soluble vitamins, electrolytes and lymphocytes [12]. In approximately 50% of conservatively treated cases, a spontaneous leak closure is achieved after varying periods of time, otherwise a surgical intervention is necessary [51, 116].

Apart from surgical injury to the thoracic duct, various other causes such as infections, neoplasms, postactinic damage, thrombosis of the jugular or subclavian veins may be responsible for the formation of a chylothorax. The two following case reports suggest possible endoscopic solutions to the problem.

11.2 Case Reports

Postoperative Chylothorax

A 69-year-old man developed a postoperative, left-sided chylothorax following a triple aorto-coronary bypass operation [87]. The patient's aortic valve had been replaced in 1977, and a first aorto-coronary bypass operation was performed at that time. Conservative therapy with thorax drainage and parenteral hyperalimentation for more than 2 weeks achieved no success. We therefore decided on a thoracoscopic approach. The chyle leak was exposed thoracoscopically following localization with lymphangio-CT and sealed successfully with fibrin glue. The previous daily loss of approximately 450 ml of chyle stopped immediately after the intervention. Postoperative X-rays revealed a fully expanded lung. Further X-rays on the first postoperative day and 6 and 12 months later showed normal conditions.

Operative Technique. Supine position, local anaesthesia, two entry sites. After complete evacuation of the chylothorax, two parasternal trocar sleeves were placed in the third intercostal space. The sites of the incisions were selected posterior to the cranial margin of the aortic arch based on the leakage of contrast medium seen on the CT scan (Fig. 35). After introducing the 0° telescope, a continuous flow of chyle drops could be seen between sail-like adhesions. The fistula could be visualized precisely. Using the injection cannula, 1 ml fibrin glue (fast-acting components) was injected into the fistula and the flow of chyle was stopped. After placing a

Fig. 36. Idiopathic
chylothorax. Parietal
pleura (*small arrow*) and
atelectatic lung (*large
arrow*)

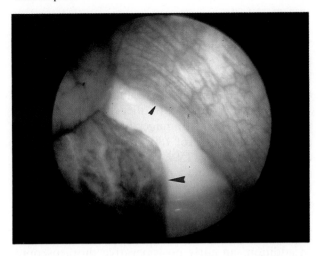

closed drain beside the sealed opening of the fistula, the
intervention was completed as usual.

Non-malignant Chylothorax of Unknown Aetiology

A woman born in 1937 was referred to us for investigation and
therapy of a recurrent, therapy-resistant and unexplained
chylothorax. Neither the medical history nor clinical investigation using various techniques was able to throw any light on
the cause of the condition. The patient remained afebrile and
was in good general health. The only symptom was restricted
respiratory function whenever the chylothorax refilled. On
thoracoscopy, no pathological changes could be found. The
endoscopic image was similar to that illustrated in Fig. 36.
With no indication of malignancy (histological frozen sections), we decided to proceed to an extensive endoscopic
parietal pleurectomy as discussed and agreed with the patient
preoperatively. The definitive histological diagnosis was re-
active mesothelial proliferation of the pleura. Postoperatively
the lung adhered to the endothoracic fascia as hoped. The
patient was discharged on the sixth postoperative day and has
remained free of symptoms since then.

Operative Technique. Lateral position, double-lumen intubation, standard entry sites. The technical procedure is as for
parietal pleurectomy (cf. Chap. 9). The sole difference is
the extension of the pleurectomy, which in this case was
continued in the basal direction into the costodiaphragmatic
recess and completed by excision of parts of the diaphrag-
matic pleura.

11.3 Conclusions

The current surgical therapy of postoperative chylothorax consists of attempting to expose and
ligate the thoracic duct [116, 129, 153]. This technique was first described by Lampson in 1948 [99].
Other reported therapeutic measures include talc
pleurodesis [2, 53], drainage by means of pleuro-
peritoneal shunts [116, 180] or intrapleural application of fibrin [3, 159]. The thoracoscopic leak
closure we performed represents a procedure of
low invasiveness which can be used immediately
following diagnosis of postoperative chylothorax.
The loss of vitamins, electrolytes and immuno-
logically important lymphocytes can be avoided.
In addition, an early postoperative thoracoscopic
intervention has the advantage that adhesions are
absent or fresh and easy to divide.

In cases of idiopathic chylothorax, thoracoscopy can fulfil two purposes. It allows a thorough
diagnostic examination of the pleural cavity (cf.
Chap. 8) and depending on the diagnosis permits
an extensive parietal pleurectomy or, in cases of
malignant disease, talc pleurodesis (cf. Chap. 17).

12 Pleural Empyema

12.1 General

When pulmonary processes exist, the equilibrium between exudation and absorption is disturbed. Massive exudation of fibrin and fibrin deposits are possible. The shallow breathing technique adopted by the patient to avoid the pain caused by these conditions further promotes the fast organization of the deposits by fibrocytes with accompanying destruction of the mesothelium and adhesions of both pleural membranes. The result is a marked restriction and even total loss of pulmonary mobility with a corresponding loss of vital capacity.

This sequence of events is most noticeable if there is bacterial infection. Not every contaminated pleural effusion develops into empyema. However if bacterial infection is present, the probability is high that it will develop [61, 78, 103, 134].

By definition, empyema is characterized by a collection of pus in the pleural cavity. The pathological development can be divided into three stages: (1) the exudative, (2) the fibrino-purulent and (3) the fibrosing, organizing stage. These stages are however not clearly demarcated and often overlap and coexist in different regions of the thoracic cavity (loculations, basal recesses).

Pleural empyema occurs in 37% of cases as a result of infection of the respiratory tract, in 33% due to a previous operation, in 10% due to an intra-abdominal source of infection, and in 10% the cause is iatrogenic [126].

If bacterial pleurisy with the danger of empyema is suspected, the evaluation of the effusion is decisive in deciding the action to be taken. If the effusion is no longer serosanguineous but viscous or if it clots quickly after being drawn off owing to a high protein content, adequate aspiration by thoracocentesis can no longer be expected and surgical intervention is necessary. When this stage is reached, cell counts, and the glucose and lactate dehydrogenase (LDH) levels are less important in terms of the prognostic evaluation [61, 78, 103, 104, 126, 134].

With the onset of the fibrinopurulent phase, sail-like adhesions form, the pleural membrane becomes adhesive and loculations are created. The process progresses to fixation and reduced pulmonary expansion. With the invasion of fibroblasts, the visceral pleura finally loses its elasticity and a "lung cortex" results [4].

What is the potential of thoracoscopy for treating pleural empyema? By dividing adhesions, loculations can be opened and the pleural cavity as a whole restored (Fig. 37). After thorough lavage a drainage system can be established.

12.2 Operative Procedure

Lateral position, double-lumen intubation. The positions of the three entry sites are selected based on the CT scan between the fourth and eighth intercostal spaces (cf. Fig. 37).

Exudative to Early Fibrinopurulent Phase (Fig. 38). The aim of the intervention is to free and examine the whole thoracic cavity, including the fissures. The 0° telescope is inserted in the fourth intercostal space after emptying the pleural cavity as far as possible. Fresh adhesions between the two pleural membranes are carefully broken through with the palpator or dissector and sail-like adhesions are divided. Once it is certain that the whole pleural cavity is free including the various recesses and the interlobal fissures, lavage is started alternately irrigating and aspirating warm Ringer's lactate, 500 ml at a time until between 4 and 5 l have been used. An apical drain is then placed through the fourth intercostal space. The dorsobasal drain is inserted through an additional

Fig. 37. a Preoperative CT scan through a pleural empyema left. **b** CT scan at the same height in the same patient after thoracoscopic adhesiolysis, débridement with the shaver and irrigation

Fig. 38. Exudative phase: fine fibrinous adhesions apical with the start of empyema formation. To obtain a view within the pleural space, the adhesions must be carefully released and divided

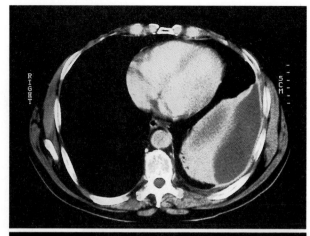

37a

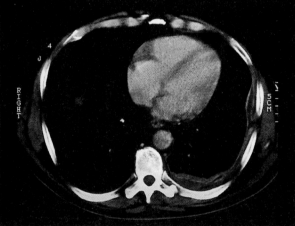

b

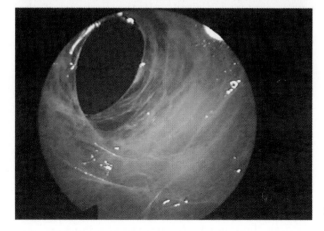

38

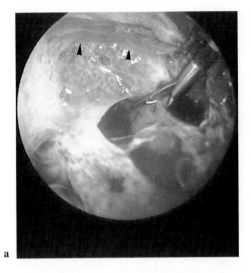

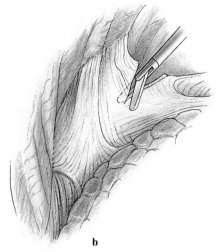

a
b

incision under optical vision and placed at the deepest point.

Fibrinopurulent Phase (Fig. 39). Lateral position, double-lumen intubation. The positions of the three entry sites are selected based on the CT scan between the fourth and eighth intercostal spaces. If the subsequent insufflation of CO_2 through the Verres needle is obstructed (cf. Sect. 3.6) it must be repeated at another location. The incision can be extended to finger size and the pleural cavity explored digitally. If the findings of the exploration are satisfactory, the thoracoscopy is continued by introducing the first trocar. Any fluid is carefully aspirated and the telescope is then inserted. The position of the second incision is decided on the basis of the endoscopic findings. Using the dissector, palpator and suction tube adhesions are divided step by step and fluid, fibrin bands and pus are evacuated by alternate irrigation and aspiration. When the space is sufficiently large to introduce the third trocar, the suction-irrigation tube is used parallel to the palpator/dissector to make dissection easier.

The fissures of the lung can be exposed after dividing their normally superficial adhesions and

Fig. 39a,b. Empyema in the fibrinopurulent stage. Loculations between the lung and thorax wall (*arrows*) are opened

Fig. 40. Endoscopic image with the shaver in action. Thorax wall, the fibrin deposits are sticking to the diaphragm. The *arrows* point into the costodiaphragmatic recess

Fig. 41a,b. Shaver for evacuating fibrin deposits in empyema. **a** Generator, motorized handle and endoscopy attachments. **b** Shaver tip in the optical field of view. The shaver must only be used with the knife pointing towards the telescope

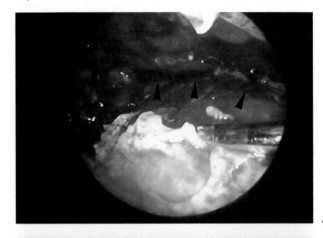

40

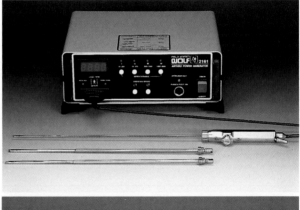

41a

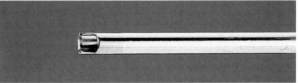

b

they serve as anatomical landmarks. Even at the early fibrinopurulent stage, the recesses (cf. Fig. 3) are usually covered by thick fibrin deposits. They must be examined, unequivocally identified, exposed with the dissector and removed with the shaver (Fig. 40). The shaver must only be used with the blade pointing towards the telescope (Fig. 41). After freeing the whole pleural cavity and removing the fibrin deposits from both pleural membranes, the lung is cautiously ventilated. It must now be seen to expand completely as far as the thoracic wall. If this is the case, drainage is established as described above and the intervention is completed. If, however, there is still a dead space between a lung with reduced elasticity and the evacuated pleural cavity and if the lung cannot be freed thoracoscopically, open decortication must be performed.

12.3 Our Own Experience

Up to now, 16 patients, six women and ten men, ranging in age from 20 to 73 years (mean 53 years) have been treated thoracoscopically by our study group. Table 13 lists the stage of the disease, the type of anaesthesia and the clinical course of events. In every case, we were able to make a visual diagnosis of the pleural cavity. In one case, decortication was performed by anterolateral

Table 13. Emphysema patients ($n = 16$)

Patient	Age (years)	Stage[a]	Anaesthesia	Success	Conversion	Second intervention	Remarks
Female	20	3	DL	−		Thoracotomy	Trapped lung
Female	50	3	Int	−	Decortication		Pannus
Male	53	3	Int	−	Fenestration		Pneumonectomy cavity
Female	53	3	DL	−		Thoracotomy	Trapped lung
Female	29	2–3	DL	+			
Female	37	2–3	DL	−	Decortication		Pannus
Male	60	2–3	DL	−		Thoracotomy	Febrile
Male	62	2–3	Int	+			
Male	70	2–3	DL	+			Preoperative septic-toxic shock
Male	73	2–3	LA	+			
Male	36	2	DL	+			
Female	54	2	DL	+			
Male	55	2	DL	+			
Male	61	2	LA	+		Second thoracoscopy	Evacuation of residual exudate
Female	65	2	DL	+			
Male	73	2	LA	+			

Int, intubation anaesthesia; DL, double-lumen intubation; LA, local anaesthesia
[a] Stages: 1, exudative; 2, fibrinopurulent, fibrosing.

Fig. 42a,b. Trapped lung after thoracoscopic evacuation of pleural empyema. Despite adequate drainage, absence of fever and normalized leukocyte counts, the lung has not expanded 7 days after the intervention. A dead space has become established. **a** X-ray **b** CT

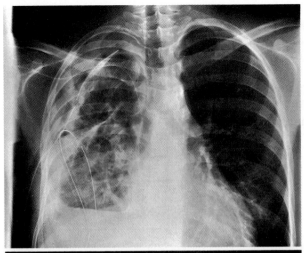

a

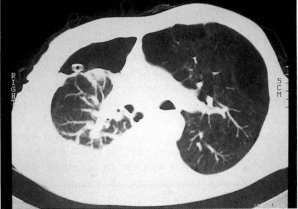

b

thoracotomy during the same session because considerable deposits were present on the visceral pleura. In one case where an empyematous pneumonectomy cavity had been left after the lung had been removed because of bronchial carcinoma, the empyema was evacuated, multiple biopsies taken and thorax fenestration performed, following which the cavity healed.

In two cases, despite the absence of fever and insignificant serous exudation, open decortication was necessary 1 week later owing to a trapped lung (Fig. 42). Due to a renewed increase of empyema discovered on X-ray and a febrile condition, an open operation was necessary in one further patient. After 5 clinically unremarkable days without fever and with dry drainage, a second thoracoscopy under local anaesthesia was performed successfully in a diabetic patient when a paravertebral encapsulated residual empyema at the level of the hilum was found on X-ray.

In 9 out of 15 cases, therefore, we were able to treat this serious condition without a thoracotomy. The operations lasted between 15 and 90 min (mean 55 min). There were no intraoperative complications. Blood transfusion was not necessary. All the patients could be extubated immediately following the intervention.

12.4 Conclusions

In the exudative to early fibrinopurulent phase of empyema, a thoracoscopic intervention can prevent the progress of the disease. Loculations can be opened under vision and their contents aspirated and adhesions can be divided. In contrast to Braimbridge's study group [80, 140, 145] we are convinced that three entry sites are necessary rather than a single site, to allow endoscopic visual control and the help of an assistant. Kaiser [95] meets the requirement of visual dissection better by using a mediastinoscope, since its diameter allows the introduction of instruments and simultaneous optical control. The operation restores the pleural cavity to a single space and allows lavage and establishment of a drainage system at the lowest point [124, 181].

In the late fibrinopurulent phase, scarring in the recesses can be evacuated with the shaver and the fresh deposits on both pleural membranes removed with the dissector. If the latter proves impossible, our experience indicates that despite a free pleural cavity, open decortication should be performed early since even when the infectious process has been stopped with a sterile pleural cavity the trapped lung can no longer expand (Fig. 42). Technically the decortication of the collapsed lung as necessary for thoracoscopy remains an unsolved problem. We have not succeeded in bursting visceral scars using high pressure as described by some authors [74, 80, 95], even at a peak inspiratory pressure of 50 mmHg.

The thoracoscopic treatment of pleural empyema has made a promising start. In terms of technique and instrumentation the procedure is still at the stage of clinical research. Immediate progress in the endoscopic treatment of this serious disease could be made if patients were referred for thoracoscopy at an earlier stage than is the case today. Organized pleural structures can often be found only 2 weeks after the first symptoms occur [4, 136].

13 Bronchopleural Fistula

13.1 General

Initial postoperative loss of air via drains following interventions involving resection of the lung is not uncommon and provided only a small quantity is lost in the first few days is only of limited clinical significance. Normally this is caused by leaking sutures where bridges of parenchyma have been divided or by circumscribed iatrogenic lesions of the visceral pleura.

Nevertheless, a bronchopleural insufficiency must always be considered. Every bronchopleural fistula carries the risk of infection and the pleural cavity must be classified as potentially contaminated. A leak also means the risk of an intrathoracic dead space being formed with a trapped section of lung. Clinically relevant bronchopleural fistulae as complications of previous operations on the lung in the form of ischaemia (denudation of the stump), insufficient sutures and early infection are therefore a serious problem in thoracic surgery.

Thoracoscopy provides various, as yet scarcely tried, possibilities of early diagnostic localization and therapy if the findings are suitable without subjecting the patient to undue strain.

13.2 Operative Procedure

The anaesthesia depends on the general condition of the patient and the respiratory situation, the extent of the fistula and the time that has elapsed since the operation which caused it. If the lung operation was performed only a few days previously, the patient shows no signs of serious infection and the amount of air escaping and radiology suggest a circumscribed process without an extensive dead space, the intervention can be performed under local anaesthesia in the supine position. The incision sites are selected according to the area in which the leak is suspected and taking into account the location of the thoracotomy scar. Even after a few days, there is already a broad adhesive band between the lung parenchyma and the inner wall of the thorax in the area of the incision. If they are divided from the intercostal space they may well bleed.

If the leak is in the area of the upper lobe the intercostal spaces three to six are suitable. To explore the area of the middle or lower lobes, the fourth to eighth intercostal spaces are more suitable. When using the basal intercostal spaces, special care is needed to avoid postoperative adhesions between the costal pleura and the diaphragm (cf. Sect. 3.9).

After careful insufflation of approximately 300 ml CO_2 gas through the Verres needle the first trocar is introduced. Gas insufflation is then continued under vision and the second entry site established (also under vision). At an insufflation pressure above 10 mmHg and/or if the flow is slow, blind insufflation is stopped and the first incision made transthoracically with the scissors.

If a dead space has been identified preoperatively by X-ray, the first trocar should be inserted into this cavity without prior gas insufflation and the cavity then explored with the 0° telescope. Dissection is started with the palpator introduced through a second incision, and space is gradually created. In the first postoperative days, broad adhesions with the exception of those in the area of the thoracotomy can be divided easily and with little risk of bleeding.

The sutures on the bronchial stump and the bridges of parenchyma are visualized with the telescope and checked. Using the jet of water and by briefly ventilating this side of the lung, it is possible to discover a leak. If a leak is found, material is taken from the area of the fistula for histological, cytological and bacteriological tests.

If the area of the leak appears on endoscopic examination to be surrounded by vital tissue, we attempt to close the leak. Depending on the site and size of the leak we either use fibrin glue (1–2 ml fast-acting) or an endosuture (Prolene, Ethicon). If the immediately surrounding area appears necrotic, débridement is performed (suction tube, scissors, punch), remembering that there are closely adjacent pulmonary vessels. If vital parenchyma can be revivified, the leak is then closed. After checking the operative correction and establishing drainage, the intervention is completed as normal.

13.3 Our Own Experience

Table 14 documents our experience up to now. In eight of eleven patients, airtight conditions and subsequent infection-free healing were achieved. In three cases involving a large dead space with an infected parenchymal margin, a thoracoscopic intervention was technically impossible. Our experience shows that decortication of a trapped lung (Fig. 42) is not feasible thoracoscopically with the current technical possibilities (cf. Chap. 12). If the clinical, radiological and laboratory parameters point to an infected postoperative bronchopulmonary fistula, a therapeutic thoracoscopy does not currently represent a viable alternative since large necrotic areas around the fistula cannot be radically excised using endoscopic methods.

13.4 Conclusions

Bronchopleural fistulas, particularly large, central fistulas, following lobectomy or pneumonectomy are a serious complication of thoracic surgery. Their incidence is between 2% and 4% [105, 119, 135]. Apart from techniques in which the fistula is closed by covering it with pericardium, chest wall muscle flaps or using the greater omentum [15, 72, 127, 128, 171], bronchoscopic techniques in animal

Table 14. Bronchopleural fistula ($n = 11$)

Patient's age[a] (years)	Diagnosis	Post-operative time (days)	Findings	Technique	Results
43	ARDS, ventilated patient with barotrauma	7	Parenchyma leak, fibrin deposits	Intraparenchymal fibrin injection	Airtight lung
64	Bronchial carcinoma, after bilobectomy	11	Leaking segmental bronchus	Fibrin injection	Airtight
76	Bronchial carcinoma, after lobectomy	14	Parenchyma leak, trapped residual lung dead space	Débridement, fibrin dispersion	Airtight 3 days, decortication because of new leak
52	Palliative lobectomy for necrotizing carcinoma	14	Trapped residual lung, empyema cavity, parenchyma leak	Débridement, fibrin injection, thoracic wall fenestration	Airtight, healed
68	Non-Hodgkin lymphoma, persistent iatrogenic pneumothorax	14	Parenchyma leak, squashy surroundings	Débridement, fibrin injection	Airtight
76	AC bypass, ventilated patient with barotrauma	5	Bullous lung, leak not found	Pleurectomy	Airtight after 12 h
59	Bronchial carcinoma after lobectomy	10	Parenchyma leak, trapped residual lung, dead space	Thoracotomy	Decortication
77	Bronchial carcinoma after lobectomy	10	Fistulous bronchus stump	Revivification, fibrin injection	Airtight
66	Bronchial carcinoma after lobectomy	12	Parenchyma leak	Fibrin injection	Airtight
59	Open decortication of the lung	14	Injured segmental bronchus	Fibrin block	Airtight 2 days, open suturing
35	Empyema with florid tuberculosis	No previous operation	Parenchyma leak, empyema	Thoracotomy	Decortication

ARDS, acute respiratory distress syndrome; AC, aortocoronary
[a] All patients were male

experiments and clinical application have been reported in recent years. In these procedures, bronchopleural fistulas were treated either by fibrin glue alone or in conjunction with a decalcified spongiosa block [59, 91, 135, 178]. There is so far only sparse literature on thoracoscopic interventions for the location and therapy of bronchopleural fistula. The diagnostic use of thoracoscopy has been reported [36, 70] and case reports of thoracoscopic treatment of fistulas by fibrin glue [21, 170], talc application [165] and using the Nd:YAG laser [21, 67] have been published.

It is too early for a detailed evaluation of the thoracoscopic method or for a comparison with bronchoscopic techniques. With the further development of suitable instruments, the thoracoscopic evaluation of a fistula, its revivification and closure with fibrin or talc, suture or stapler should represent a promising alternative to open surgery, particularly in patients with a poor overall condition. It is, however, important to tackle fistulas before clinical symptoms of a massive bronchial stump insufficiency become apparent and while evidence of the formation of pleural empyema is absent. With the low invasiveness of the intervention, we consider it justified after a waiting period of 5–7 days, and in view of the intrapleural conditions with only light adhesions it represents a technically promising approach.

14 Sympathectomy

14.1 General

Arterial vessels in a terminal flow region, as represented by the digital arteries, are not accessible to reconstructive surgery. If conservative therapy fails in primary and secondary Raynaud's syndrome, a different therapeutic technique must be applied. One possibility is thoracic sympathectomy. Hyperhidrosis of the hands or axilla with recurrent sudoriparous abscesses is also an indication for thoracic sympathectomy. The second to fifth sympathetic ganglia are responsible for the innervation of the hand and the third ganglion for the axilla. The operation can be performed endoscopically, thereby avoiding a thoracotomy.

14.2 Operative Procedure

Lateral position, double-lumen intubation, three standard entry sites. If a bilateral operation is planned under the same anaesthesia, the position is as shown in Fig. 43.

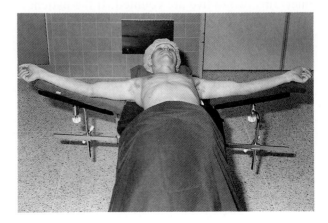

Fig. 43. Position for bilateral thoracic sympathectomy in one session

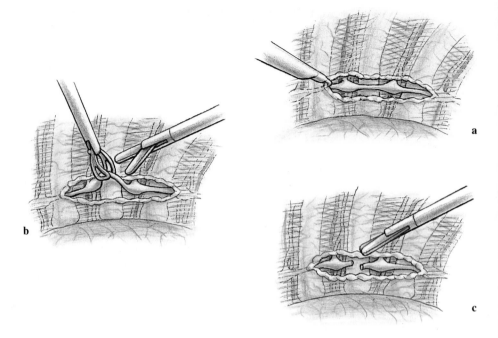

The sympathetic trunk runs on both sides of the vertebral column somewhat lateral to the heads of the ribs and extends from the base of the skull to the coccyx (cf. Figs. 1 and 4). If it is not visible owing to subpleural fat, it can be felt as a firm elastic cord which can be pushed backwards and forwards. After identifying the second rib (the first can be seen at the roof of the thoracic inlet) ribs two to five are counted. If the patient is supine, the lung is held away with a grasping forceps; in the lateral position, it falls out of the field of view itself. The parietal pleura is first incised by raising it with the coagulation probe (Fig. 44a). The trunk is then exposed and raised carefully between the ganglia (Fig. 44b). After exact definition of the ganglia to be resected, they are dissected along with their connections to the intercostal nerves (rami communicantes) using the monopolar coagulation probe or scissors (Fig. 44c). Care is necessary to avoid damaging the intercostal nerves; otherwise unpleasant dysaesthesia

Fig. 44. a Incision of the pleura above the sympathetic trunk. **b** Raising the trunk. **c** Dividing the sympathetic trunk. This is followed by excision of the ganglia by dividing the connections to the intercostal nerves (rami communicantes)

may result (cf. Chap. 4). Care is also required to avoid the veins crossing the sympathetic trunk. These are particularly large on the right hand side where they come together before joining the azygos vein. Bleeding from these veins is difficult to control endoscopically. Coagulation is almost impossible owing to the structure of the walls, and the application of a clip or suture is also difficult owing to their central anatomical position. If there is any doubt about haemostasis and if bleeding is heavy close to the confluence, the lung must be inflated to act as a tamponade, and a transaxillary thoracotomy performed to stop the bleeding by open methods. The resected section of the sympathetic trunk is retained for histological verification and the intervention completed as usual. Immediately following the operation, a warm, dry and hyperaematized hand is the visible confirmation of an effective sympathectomy.

14.3 Our Own Experience

Some 13 patients, six women and seven men, aged between 25 and 74 years (mean 41.6 years) underwent surgery (three of them had bilateral interventions). The indications, operating time, duration of drainage and hospitalization and complications are shown in Table 15.

Except in those cases where a hyperhidrosis was manifest, sympathectomy was preceded by the angiological tests listed in Table 16 to reinforce the diagnosis in cases of circulatory disturbance.

14.4 Conclusions

If a thoracic sympathectomy is indicated, it can be performed with relative ease thoracoscopically, which subjects the patient to far less strain. A thoracotomy is now only indicated when the pleural cavity is completely obliterated. While long-term results are absent for the other thoracoscopic interventions, Wittmoser [188–192] and Wepf [46] have proved the efficiency and low com-

Table 15. Thoracoscopic sympathectomy

Patient	Age (years)	Indication	Operating time (min)	Drainage time (h)	Postoperative hospitalization (days)	Complications	Sympathectomy effect
Male	55	Critical ischaemia, fourth digit with ulnar artery occlusion	45	25	4	None	+ +
Male	47	Raynaud's disease with hypothenar hammer syndrome	50	24	4	None	+ +
Male	25	Posttraumatic Raynaud's disease	40	24	1	None	+ +
Male	55	Microemboli with spurious aneurysm, subclavian artery	30	24	2	None	+ +
Male	29	Hyperhidrosis, bilateral	35 right 30 left	24 24	2	None None	+ + + +
Male	40	Microemboli with spurious aneurysm, subclavian artery	65	48	11	Thoracotomy due to bleeding intercostal vein	
Male	52	Raynaud's disease	40	No drain	3	Terminated due to obliterated pleural cavity	−
Female	74	Critical ischaemia, unknown aetiology	40	24	3	None	+
Female	49	Microangiopathy with diabetes mellitus	40	1	2	None	+
Female	32	Hyperhidrosis with recurrent spiradenitis, bilateral	30 right 30 left	24 24	1	None	+ +
Female	46	Iatrogenic critical ischaemia after embolization of an A-V deformity	30	24	3	None	+ +
Female	29	Sclerodermatitis	50 right 35 left	24 48	2 3	None None	+ + + +
Female	43	Ergotism	25	24	2	None	+ +

A total of 16 sympathectomies were performed in 13 patients
A-V, arteriovenous

Table 16. Preoperative examinations prior to elective thoracoscopic sympathectomy

---

Anamnesis and clinical examination
Cold exposure test
Occlusion pressure measurements on all four extremities
Ten finger oscillogram
Capillary microscopy
Laboratory tests:
    White and red blood count
    Blood sedimentation reaction
    Anti-nuclear antibodies
    Rheumatoid factors
Conventional X-ray of affected hand in two planes
If microangiopathy is suspected: digital, intra-arterial subtraction angiography

---

plication rate of thoracoscopic sympathectomy over a long period and in several hundred patients. With adequate experience and with the consent of the patient, the intervention can also be undertaken on an outpatient basis without involving any inordinate risks [46]. Possible intraoperative risks and complications such as injury to intercostal vessels or nerves or damage to the cervicothoracic ganglion with consequent Horner's syndrome can be avoided with adequate care and training.

14.5 Other Methods

As an alternative to surgical resection of the sympathetic trunk, Toomes and Linder [163] describe superficial coagulation of the pleural area around the second to fourth ganglia. Pneumologists perform a sympathicolysis by instilling sclerosing agents into the subpleural space beside the nerves. Only two incisions are necessary for this technique which is performed under local infiltration anaesthesia combined with i.v. sedation [65, 66].

15 Resection of Cysts and Tumours in the Thoracic Cavity

15.1 Extrathoracic Tumours

Introduction

A shadow found by chance on the chest X-ray is cause for concern for both doctor and patient, even when the location, form and extent strongly suggest a benign lesion. If growth of the tumour can be determined retrospectively or in the period following the discovery, not only verification by biopsy is indicated but also resection of the process. Surgical thoracoscopy is a suitable, definitive therapeutic method, which allows not only verification of the diagnosis by biopsy but also resection and evacuation.

Operative Procedure

Lateral position, double-lumen intubation. The preliminary entry sites are selected based on the radiological findings. CT scans are particularly suitable in this respect (Fig. 45a). After the initial overall visual examination, the lesion is palpated with the rod to determine the size, consistency and mobility of the tumour on the underlying tissue (Fig. 45b). The resection is started by incising the pleura with the coagulation hook (Fig. 45c). The vessels supplying the tumour are coagulated or occluded with a clip (Fig. 45d).

To avoid any risk of contamination of the thoracic wall by the tumour, it is always extracted in a plastic sack. While the intercostal muscles can usually be forced apart, extension of the skin incision may be necessary depending on the size of the specimen. After irrigation of the operating field and a careful check to ensure haemostasis, the operation is completed as usual.

Fig. 45. a CT scan: paravertebral intrathoracic neurilemoma located behind the aorta in a patient with Recklinghausen's disease. b The neurilemoma (diameter 3.5 cm) is located on top of the aorta. The eighth rib can be seen at 11 o'clock. c To release the neurilemoma, the parietal pleura is incised with the coagulation hook. d Released from its surroundings, the neurilemoma is suspended solely by the vessel-nerve pedicle which is clipped before it is divided

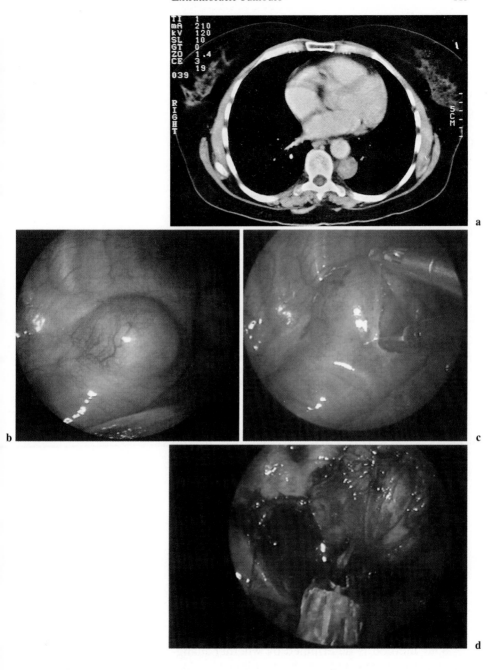

Our Own Experience

Intrathoracic Neurilemoma. (Fig. 45a–d). A 57-year-old female patient known to have Recklinghausen's disease was referred to the neurosurgical department of the University Hospital Bern owing to thoracic pain. The diagnostic tests revealed an intrathoracic neurilemoma at the height of T8. Resection was indicated owing to the painful symptoms and to exclude malignant degeneration of the suspected neurilemoma. The intervention lasted 60 min; drainage could be stopped 24 h after the operation. The patient was discharged 4 days later free of pain.

Intrathoracic Lipoma [55]. In a 45-year-old, obese female patient a left-sided, parietal shadow had been found on the chest X-ray (Fig. 46a). The CT scan led to the diagnosis of a suspected lipoma originating from the parietal pleura (Fig. 46b). Owing to the clear growth of the lesion and the recent development of a cough, the patient was referred to our department for resection of the tumour.

The chest X-ray on admittance confirmed the existence of a probably benign pleural tumour. After tests the dry cough was interpreted as asthmatic in character and not due to the pleural findings. Thoracoscopic exploration revealed the expected lipoma (Fig. 46c). The tumour could be removed in toto without difficulty. Histology confirmed that the lipoma was benign. The thorax drain placed intraoperatively was removed on the first postoperative day. Following further pneumological diagnostic tests, the patient was discharged 6 days later.

Conclusions

Intrathoracic cysts and tumours represent a fruitful area of activity for minimally invasive techniques. In 1985, Faurschou described thoracoscopy as a diagnostic possibility for evaluating thoracic wall processes on the basis of seven cases [50]. Greschuchna published an overview on the same lines in 1989 [62]. The atlas of thoracoscopy by Brandt and Loddenkemper [26, 27] lists reports of successful evacuation and necrotization of intrathoracic cysts [23, 77, 96, 112, 137, 155, 161]. Only recently the successful video-thoracoscopic resection of a bronchogenic cyst was also described [122].

Our method is determined by whether malignancy is to be expected, i.e. by oncological guidelines. If malignancy is suspected, the specimen removed is sent for frozen section in its plastic sack. If the suspicion is confirmed, we convert to

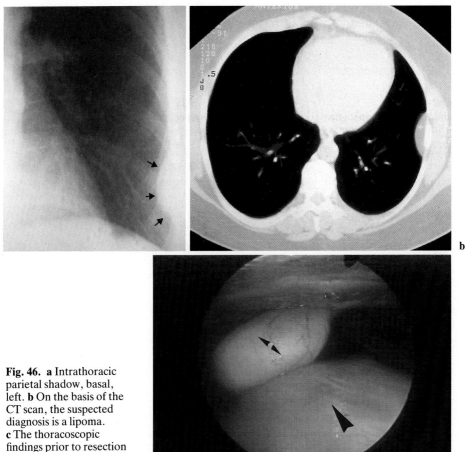

Fig. 46. a Intrathoracic parietal shadow, basal, left. **b** On the basis of the CT scan, the suspected diagnosis is a lipoma. **c** The thoracoscopic findings prior to resection (*small arrows* lipoma, *large arrow* diaphragm)

an open operation if this is indicated oncologically and is justifiable in terms of respiratory risk.

15.2 Intrapulmonary Tumours

Introduction
With the currently available instruments and techniques (ligature, stapler, sharp dissection of the parenchyma followed by application of fibrin sealant), it is possible to take large pulmonary biopsies. For peripheral, circumscribed lesions, which cannot be conclusively evaluated cytologically or histologically with existing non-invasive diagnostic techniques, thoracoscopy is a useful method for obtaining a reliable diagnosis (cf. Chap. 8). This is the case in approximately 20%–25% of patients with bronchial carcinoma where, despite the variety of options (transbronchial or percutaneous fine-needle biopsy, brush cytology, sputum cytology, etc.), a reliable diagnosis is not possible without thoracotomy [157].

After preoperative localization of the tumour by CT scan, thoracotomy can be replaced by thoracoscopy providing the lesion is located peripherally and the biopsy taken by wedge resection. By taking only a small peritumorous section of parenchyma, this intervention can even be performed in patients with impaired pulmonary and cardiac functions. In our series of over 250 patients, of which 23% were older than 65 years, all could be extubated immediately after the intervention.

Even when a histological diagnosis is possible, the non-resectability can only be demonstrated at thoracotomy in 3%–25% of tumour patients [1, 147, 157]. Small metastatic nodules on the pleura and tumour infiltration in surrounding structures such as the vena cava, oesophagus, and vertebral bodies (cf. Figs. 1 and 4) cannot always be recognized by the imaging techniques. These patients can profit from a diagnostic thoracoscopy performed prior to a planned thoracotomy under the same anaesthesia.

If a thoracotomy must be ruled out for respiratory reasons, and if the solitary tumour is peripheral and the CT of the mediastinum is unremarkable (clinically a T1N0M0 patient), thoracoscopic wedge resection should be considered as a therapeutic measure and prospectively evaluated. As far as we are aware, there are only isolated publications describing wedge resection for the removal of bronchial carcinomas via thoracotomy which could be used for comparison [47].

Operative Technique

The operative technique is identical to that of pulmonary wedge resection as described in Chap. 9. Preliminary entry sites suited to the location of the pathological findings are selected with the aid of CT scans. Freeing the pulmonary ligament and mobilizing the lung in the basal sections presents no problem thoracoscopically. Intraoperatively, care must be taken that the tumour in the resected wedge is surrounded on all sides by healthy lung parenchyma (Fig. 47c,d). The specimen must be removed in a plastic bag. The local radical excision must be confirmed by frozen section. If these conditions are met, the intervention can be completed in the usual way.

Our Own Experience

Case Report 1. During treatment of a female patient for ulcers caused by circulatory disorders, a peripheral pulmonary tumour was discovered in the latero-basal segment of the right lower lobe (Fig. 47a,b). Respiratory function tests prohibited thoracotomy in this obese patient. For this reason, and in the absence of suspicious mediastinal lymph nodes on the CT scan, we decided to resect the tumour thoracoscopically. It was possible to resect the tumour within healthy tissue both macroscopically and microscopically (Fig. 47c,d). There were no postoperative complications and the patient was able to return to the dermatological department 4 days later.

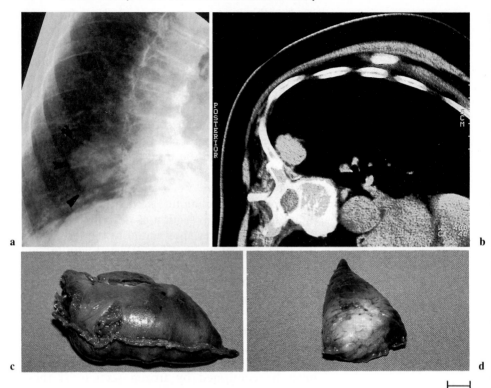

1 cm

Case Report 2. Bronchoscopy and fine-needle biopsy under CT control failed to provide a diagnosis of a fast-growing coin lesion in the anterior and superior segment of the lingula of the right upper lobe of a 38-year-old male patient. Owing to the short anamnesis and the rapid growth of the tumour, a small-cell bronchial carcinoma could not be excluded by differential diagnosis. The intraoperative frozen section of the tumour removed thoracoscopically from healthy tissue produced the diagnosis of a moderately differentiated squamous cell carcinoma, as a result of which the intervention was extended to a lobectomy of the upper lobe and formal mediastinal lymph node dissection. This allowed histological confirmation of the preoperative CT staging as T1N0M0.

Case Report 3. A 74-year-old male patient was suffering from bilateral tumours. The centrally located tumour on the left was diagnosed as a squamous cell carcinoma. The solitary, peripheral tumour in the latero-basal segment of the right lower lobe was not accessible for fine-needle biopsy owing to its small diameter (<1 cm) and a thoracoscopic resection was undertaken. After an intraoperative search with the palpator and parenchyma forceps lasting 30 min, the tumour was located and resected in healthy tissue. It also proved to be a

Fig. 47. a A right-sided paravertebral coin lesion on the semilateral radiograph. **b** CT scan of the same findings. **c** Specimen taken during thoracoscopy. The tumour has been resected using the stapler (Endo-GIA 30). **d** The specimen has been opened – a bronchial carcinoma (squamous cell carcinoma)

squamous cell carcinoma. Resection of the upper lobe was performed on the left side 5 days later.

Case Report 4. A 78-year-old patient was referred to hospital because of unexplained hypertonia. In the course of the diagnostic tests, a coin lesion was found in the right upper obe. Transbronchial cytology resulted in the diagnosis of an adenocarcinoma. In the absence of evidence of distant metastasis, thoracoscopic resection was indicated owing to the advanced age of the patient. Macroscopically surrounded in toto by healthy lung parenchyma, the tumour could be removed by thoracoscopic wedge resection. Apart from retention of urine, the postoperative phase was uneventful. The patient was discharged 10 days after the intervention.

Conclusions

Thoracoscopic pulmonary wedge resection is a major extension of the diagnostic possibilities of thoracic surgery and pneumology. Peripheral tumours with an inconclusive or incomplete cytological evaluation can be removed in this way in toto.

The therapeutic use of thoracoscopic wedge resection in patients with risk factors prohibiting thoracotomy and in the absence of evidence of local, regional or systemic metastasis represents a promising curative procedure which must, however, first be subjected to a precise prospective evaluation.

From an operative/technical point of view, the localization of small intrapulmonary tumours surrounded subpleurally by a margin of parenchyma is currently the major problem. With calm and systematic intraoperative palpation of the lung while working in a comfortable position and basing the search on CT scans, we have so far been able to identify the pathology in all cases. In the near future, endoscopic ultrasound techniques will almost certainly play a major role and open up new perspectives in the surgical treatment of metastasis.

16 Pericardial Fenestration

16.1 General

The treatment of pericardial effusion as it becomes chronic depends on the basic disease and on the symptoms arising from the effusion. Whether or not malignancy is involved is fundamental to the choice of therapy. If there is no response to initial anti-inflammatory therapy with non-steroid drugs under intensive clinical observation and following all non-invasive diagnostic methods such as electro-cardiography and echocardiography, the next diagnostic step is electrocardiographically controlled puncture. If this produces negative or inconclusive results, a subxiphoid open biopsy follows.

A wide selection of therapeutic techniques exist. The range extends from conservative concepts, pericardiocentesis [30], thoracoscopic pericardial fenestration [175] and open, subxiphoid pericardiotomy as far as radical pericardectomy [106].

Thoracoscopic pericardial fenestration is one method which allows both a diagnostic (inspection, sampling of effusion, precise biopsy) and therapeutic approach to pericardial effusions at the same time.

16.2 Operative Procedure [86]

Lateral position, general, double-lumen anaesthesia, three standard incisions. Induction of the pneumothorax is followed by a general inspection of the thoracic cavity and biopsy of any athological findings. The exterior of the pericardium is examined and the phrenic nerve identified. Depending on the course of this nerve, the fenestration is planned either ventral or dorsal to it. The pericardium is grasped carefully with an atraumatic forceps and raised. After incising the pericardium with scissors, the effusion is carefully aspirated and sent for bacteriological, cytological and chemical examination. Care must be taken not to apply suction to the epicardium to avoid cardiac dysrhythmia. Isolated supraventricular extrasystoles caused by contact with the heart during the intervention are nevertheless practically unavoidable. After opening the pericardium, a suitably sized flap is created (Fig. 48). The fenestration is completed by a thorough check to ensure complete haemostasis. Through the opening, the corresponding half of the pericardial cavity can be probed with the angled blunt palpator and adhesions located. It is also possible to introduce the rigid or an additional endoscope to explore the pericardial sac. The intervention is terminated as usual.

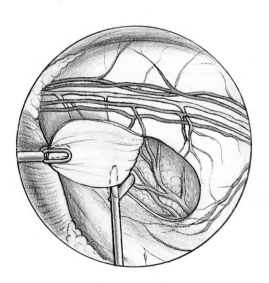

Fig. 48. Pericardial fenestration

16.3 Our Own Experience

Case Report 1. A 45-year-old female was referred for diagnostic and therapeutic pericardial fenestration owing to persistent pericardial effusion and thickening of the pericardium in conjunction with cardiomegaly of unknown aetiology already diagnosed in 1980. Intraoperatively, 300 ml of effusion (cytology and bacteriology negative) were evacuated and a 44 cm pericardial window was created (histology: chronic connective tissue proliferation). There were no postoperative complications. The drain could be removed after 24 h with the lung expanded; postoperative hospitalization lasted 3 days. Eleven months later, the patient had no symptoms and required no medication, the cardiac silhouette on the chest X-ray was unremarkable for the patient's age and the echocardiograph was normal.

Case Report 2. A 64-year-old male had undergone resection of the left upper lobe in 1984 after discovery of a pulmonary adenocarcinoma. On 9 April 1991, a pericardial effusion had to be punctured as an emergency measure owing to acute cardiac tamponade. Cytology of the effusion revealed adenocarcinomatous cells consistent with the pulmonary carcinoma of 1984. Owing to a renewed increase in effusion, thoracoscopic pericardial fenestration was performed on the 1 May. The preoperative CT scan showed a thickening of the bronchial walls of the left lower lobe, the pericardium and extensive areas of the pleura. Owing to the existing thickening of the pleura on the left side, the palliative pericardial fenestration was performed on the right. Intraoperatively more than 500 ml of blood-tinged effusion was evacuated. After making a T-shaped incision, parts of the pericardium were removed to leave a window approximately 5 × 4 cm. Postoperative drainage lasted 24 h and the patient was discharged after 4 days. Two months later, the patient had no symptoms originating from the heart, and no cardiomegaly could be determined radiologically.

Case Report 3. In a 65-year-old patient with recurrent myopericarditis, the echocardiogram revealed liquid areas. To confirm the diagnosis, a left-sided thoracoscopic pericardial biopsy was planned. The endoscopic examination showed that the movement of the pericardium was synchronous with the action of the heart. The thickened pericardium could not be grasped with the endoscopic forceps, and an open transthoracic perimyocardial biopsy was necessary. In the area visible, the pericardial sac was completely obliterated. The histological diagnosis was a non-specific active fibrinous constrictive pericarditis. One month later an open periepicardectomy was performed for hypokinesis of the trapped right ventricle.

16.4 Conclusions

The timing of the therapeutic intervention is dictated primarily by the clinical symptoms. The quantity of effusion is not of primary importance, but rather the time in which it accumulates. If the rate of increase is high, this can result in an acute tamponade [52]. The decision to operate is supported by the echocardiographical findings. With thoracoscopy, it is not only possible to perform paracentesis of recurrent pericardial effusions under vision, but also to establish a comprehensive diagnosis with extensive examination and specific biopsy of pathological processes [108, 157]. The accuracy can be compared with that of open biopsy, which is over 90% for pericardial effusions resulting from malignancy [98]. Without subjecting the patient to unwarranted strain, thoracoscopic pericardial fenestration can bring about fast and effective alleviation of symptoms, even in cases of advanced malignancy when the general condition of the patient is very poor.

The standard entry site should be in the left of thorax which is anatomically more suitable. Injury to the phrenic nerve when making the incision in the pericardium can be avoided by identifying the nerve unequivocally before dissection. If the left pleural cavity is obliterated (see *Case Report 2*), entry is possible through the right thoracic cavity. Fenestration of the pericardial sac from the right of the thorax is, however, difficult for a number of reasons and not without danger. The pericardium does not protrude like a balloon but is flat. The surface available is not as large as on the left. The right atrium below is difficult to distinguish from the bluish shimmering pericardium through the thoracoscope or on the monitor. Injury to the thin atrium wall is therefore an attendant risk.

Despite free access to the pericardium, effusive constrictive pericarditis can make thoracoscopic incision and fenestration impossible, since the thickening of the pericardium prevents it from being grasped and raised. As described in *Case Report 3*, the endoscopic method is then no longer a safe alternative to open pericardial biopsy

despite echocardiographical diagnosis and localization of effusions.

Apart from video thoracoscopy, the literature
also includes descriptions of techniques in which a
so-called operating thoracoscope is used for pericardial fenestration. With one incision, this allows
both optical viewing and the introduction of instruments through a channel in the thoracoscope
[26, 27]. A promising method of pericardial and
epicardial exploration was recently described by
Maisch and Drude [111]. After filling the pericardial sac with a crystalline solution, the pericardial space can be examined via a subxiphoid
entry site. Precise inspection and specific biopsies
of the pericardium and epicardium are then
possible.

17 Therapy of Malignant Effusions

17.1 General

In patients aged over 60 years, malignant disease is the cause of exudative pleural effusions in more than 50% of cases [118]. The formation of malignant pleural effusions can be expected during the course of the disease in 26%–49% of patients with carcinoma of the breast, 10%–24% with bronchial carcinoma, 16%–17% with ovarian carcinoma and 7%–15% with malignant lymphomas [35, 75]. The pleural cavity is almost always infiltrated by tumour cells, which in can be confirmed diagnostically in more than half the cases by the cytological examination of aspirated fluid. The effusion results either from increased capillary permeability owing to distended or destroyed capillary endothelium or is caused by tumorous lymph drainage [75]. It is also not uncommon for a hypalbuminaemia in cachectic patients to be the sole or contributive cause of pleural effusions. In over 80% of cases, both pleural membranes are involved in the exudation [75, 100, 146].

Malignant pleural effusions often cause shortness of breath, coughing and thoracic pain. The clinical examination leads to a suspected diagnosis based on weakened breathing sounds, a dull percussion note and reduced respiratory mobility of the diaphragm. Fluid can be detected on X-rays in the posteroanterior (PA) view when there is more than $175\,cm^3$, or in the lateral view with as little as $100\,cm^3$ [5, 72, 132, 193]. The symptoms arising from the effusion are often the first indications of disease. They are the dominant cause of the patient feeling ill and further restrict the quality of life of this group of tumour patients whose prognosis is already extremely poor. The survival time

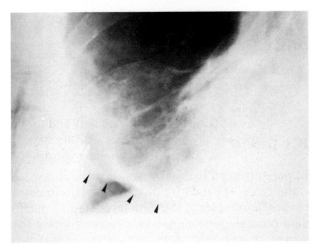

Fig. 49. After evacuating
a malignant effusion, the
trapped base of the lung
can be seen on X-ray
(*arrows*). Pleurodesis
with an established dead
space is pointless since
adhesion of the pleural
membranes is impossible

after diagnosis of malignant effusion is usually less
than 1 year [35, 144].

   After excluding the possibility of successful
systemic oncological therapy, the aim of any treatment must be fast, effective and lasting alleviation
of the respiratory symptoms. The therapeutic
strategies must be orientated towards the patho-
physiological features of the disease. The obliteration of the pleural cavity with chemical pleurodesis
by local instillation of sclerosing substances is the
most common method, but has recurrence rates of
up to 30% [21, 54]. Thoracoscopic pleurodesis
was first proposed by Béthune in France in 1935
and is still mainly propagated today in French-
speaking countries. Guérin and Boniface have a
series of 792 cases, 630 malignant and 162 non-
neoplastic effusions. They report no recurrences
in 90% of cases [16, 63]. The results of Boutin in
Marseilles are equally impressive, with personal
experience of 300 cases of malignant effusion and
a success rate of over 90% after talc pleurodesis
[21]. Boutin also reviews the literature covering a
total of 1244 patients treated with talc pleurodesis
with an average success rate of 87%.

   The success of pleurodesis depends primarily
on the careful evaluation of the patient [18].
Not all patients with malignant effusions can be

treated by thoracoscopic pleurodesis. The following conditions must be met when the therapy
is commenced:

1. The compressed lung must be shown clinically
   and radiologically to be fully expanded following drainage of the effusion (Fig. 49).

2. The evacuation of the pleural cavity and the de-
   compression of the lung must lead to a significant alleviation of the respiratory symptoms.

17.2 Operative Procedure

We keep to the guidelines of interventional thoracoscopy, as devised and recommended by pneumologists [16, 21]. The only difference is that we use
video thoracoscopy, the method we know best.
Two points of entry are normally sufficient. The
positioning of the patient must take into consideration the respiratory situation of the patient. If
there is dyspnoea or orthopnoea, the pleurodesis
can be performed with the patient in the semi-
sitting position (cf. Sect. 3.4). Local anaesthesia
combined with sedation is almost always adequate,
although in cases of chronic effusion, there is
a thickening of the pleura and correspondingly
reduced sensitivity to pain; pleural pain caused

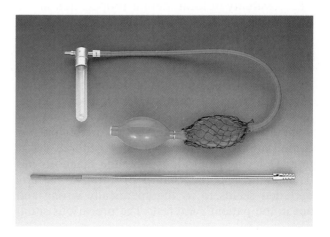

Fig. 50. Boutin's powder
atomizer

by the strongly hyperosmotic talc particles must, therefore, be taken into consideration. Sterile talcum powder (not more than 10 ml) is sprayed with a talc atomizer (Fig. 50) and distributed on the parietal and visceral pleura under vision as homogeneously as possible. The thoracic drain remains in position for a maximum of 3–4 days.

17.3 Our Own Experience

Between January 1990, when we introduced operative thoracoscopy, and February 1992, we performed thoracoscopy for pleurodesis in 42 patients. In eleven cases, we used fibrin glue (6 ml Tissucol, with fast-acting components). This was sprayed into the pleural cavity through a four-lumen catheter and dispersed under vision. In 31 patients, we performed talc pleurodesis.

17.4 Conclusions

The possible complications of thoracoscopic talc pleurodesis are those inherent in thoracoscopy and are generally not dangerous. They include surface lung injuries when inducing the pneumo-thorax, slight bleeding of the thoracic wall and local infection. In the large series of Boutin and Guérin, these complications are hardly mentioned since they are obviously clinically unimportant. The possibility of local tumour propagation in the area of the thoracoscopic entry site is known and occurs primarily with pleural mesothelioma [21, 33, 113, 144]. We experienced this complication in one patient with a pleural carcinosis resulting from an ipsilateral bronchial carcinoma. Thora-coscopically guided pleurodesis represents an effective first treatment and can be performed as a minimally invasive intervention involving few complications in patients in poor general condition. Delaying pleurodesis after the diagnosis has been made and the chance of curative therapy excluded seems to us therapeutically wrong and not in the patient's interest. The precarious situation of the patient is normally made worse by the rapidly developing symptoms which further diminish the patient's already short life expectancy. The loss of protein caused by the effusion increases the catabolic metabolic condition. The chance of successful adhesion becomes worse day by day owing to the growth of the tumour, the formation of loculations and thickening of the visceral pleura with a trapped lung.

18 Helpful Hints

Patient Positioning

Radiolucent Operating Table. The patient should be positioned on a radiolucent table. Although not required often, it is advisable to have the possibility of intraoperative visualization of the thorax with an image intensifier.

Position of the Upper Arm. The patient's upper arm must not be raised above the height of the shoulder on the side being operated on. Otherwise the manoeuvrability of the instruments and telescopes cephalad is restricted and therefore diminishes the view and manipulations in the basal areas of the thoracic cavity.

Intraoperative Thoracotomy. The sterile drapes must be arranged so that a fast change to a large thoracotomy is possible at any time. The necessary instruments must be close at hand.

Anaesthesia

Intubation Anaesthesia. In thoracoscopic surgery, the use of a double-lumen tube is the golden standard. It allows the operator to work with open trocar sleeves with the lung excluded from ventilation.

If a double-lumen tube cannot be used, endotracheal intubation anaesthesia with spontaneous respiration should be attempted. As with local anaesthesia, this technique allows at least a partial pneumothorax to be maintained without counterpressure caused by ventilation.

Local Anaesthesia. If the thoracoscopy is performed under local anaesthesia, the operator must not forget that careless contact with the parietal pleura and the mediastinum can cause severe pain. Traction on the lung can stimulate the vagus nerve and cause coughing; touching the heart can trigger cardiac dysrhythmia such as supraventricular extrasystoles, sinus tachycardia and vasovagal reactions.

Anxiety of Patients Under Local Anaesthesia. It is not uncommon for the locally anaesthetized patient to experience anxiety when the pneumothorax is induced, and this must be recognized by the surgeon and anaesthetist. While the surgeon stops further gas insufflation or even reverses the pneumothorax in extreme cases, the anaesthetist must evaluate the clinical somatic relevance of the situation and provide psychological support and, if necessary, resort to medical measures to calm the patient.

Operating Technique

Operative Procedure. Endoscopic surgery demands calm and well-planned action on the part of the operator when positioning the telescopes and performing dissection. "Brisk" operating is liable to become overhasty and uncontrolled owing to the magnification achieved by the telescope and since the video image is two-dimensional and the depth of focus absent, this is not without danger.

Posture of the Operator. A comfortable working position has a positive influence on the operation. The height of the table should be adjusted so that the hands can guide the instruments while remaining relaxed, and the monitor should be at eye level and directly facing the operator.

First Assistant. The first assistant should be familiar both with the anatomy and the operating technique. This allows calm positioning and guidance of the telescope. Ideally, the team should be so well versed that each is capable of performing the intervention.

Instrument Nurse. The instrument nurse must have a clear view of the monitor. This allows him or her to participate actively, anticipating the instrument changes complicated by cables and tubes.

Arrangement of Units. The devices and units should be arranged so that the circulating nurse has access to them and can operate them without encroaching on the sterile area.

Thoracoscopic Palpation. Thoracoscopic palpation can be learnt. Experience of the open thorax – anatomical structures and their consistency, features and relationship to underlying structures – must be recalled from memory and associated with the endoscopic palpation. With increasing experience, there is a synthesis between "surgical and endoscopic" palpatory sensation.

Searching for Intrapulmonary Findings. The palpation of small intrapulmonary tumours can be difficult. A systematic method, calm and patience are important. The localization made on the CT scan changes when the lung is collapsed, and this must not be forgotten when palpating.

Venous Bleeding. If venous bleeding cannot be stopped thoracoscopically and an open intervention becomes necessary, ventilating the lungs with a high average respiratory pressure can have the effect of a tamponade, preventing greater blood loss while the thoracotomy is performed.

Obliteration of the Pleural Cavity. Prior to a thoracoscopy, possible causes which could lead to pleural obliteration must be precisely investigated and searched for so that suitable patient positioning and entry sites can be planned and an unnecessary attempt at thoracoscopy can be avoided. If the information gained from a thorough medical history and clinical and radiological examinations is not unequivocal, a CT scan can often be helpful since careful study can reveal even slight thickening of the pleura.

First Incision. With the patient in the lateral position, the standard position, the first incision in the fourth intercostal space at the anterior margin of the latissimus dorsi muscle has proved best. This point provides an optimum view throughout the whole thoracic cavity. The further incisions are then always made under endoscopic vision. Their locations depend on the pathology and the intended intervention.

Previous Thoracotomy. If the patient has undergone a previous thoracotomy, thick, band-like adhesions between the inner thorax wall and the lung in the area of the scar must always be expected. These may bleed significantly from both sides depending on their age.

Lung Fissures. As an aid to anatomical orientation, lung fissures can be used. Adhesions in the fissures are normally only superficial.

Unwanted Expansion of the Lung During Suction. To avoid the unwanted expansion of the lung when using the suction tube, insufflation of CO_2 must be synchronized with the aspiration, or a trocar must be left open.

Water Test. The carefully ventilated lung is pushed section by section below the surface of instilled Ringer's solution. Air leaks can be detected using this method.

Application of Fibrin Glue Through a Reusable Cannula. The cannula must be thoroughly cleaned in Ringer's solution to prevent irreversible reduction of the lumen by dried fibrin glue. It is better to use a disposable two-lumen catheter. Its tip can be guided endoscopically with the mini grasping forceps.

Rows of Staples. If these are fired with the lung completely collapsed, our experience has shown that too strong a ventilation of the lung can lead to small tears in the visceral pleura. To prevent this, the suture can be performed on the lung when it is only partially collapsed and the lung then carefully re-inflated. In particular with emphysematous lung tissue, it is advisable to seal the suture with fast-acting fibrin glue.

Inducing the Pneumothorax

If it is not possible to induce a pneumothorax, a mini-incision can be made to allow local digital palpation of the pleural space before deciding to abandon the intervention or converting to thoracotomy. With this digital palpation, the experienced operator can distinguish between old and/or thick bands and delicate adhesions or a currently organizing pannus. With the latter two findings, a circumscribed cavity can be formed with the finger. After placing a tight skin suture with single knots, two adjacent trocars are installed in which the telescope and an instrument can be introduced. The pleural space can then be freed of adhesions step by step. At the same time, the lung is collapsed by CO_2 insufflation. This method is only suitable in double-lumen intubated patients.

Gas Insufflation. A high pressure on the scale and a slow flow rate can indicate that adhesions have formed compartments, there is partial obliteration or the needle tip is positioned incorrectly. On the other hand, if the CO_2 partial pressure of the breath rises on the capnograph at the same time as the gas insufflation, the Verres needle is probably in lung parenchyma and must be repositioned.

Adhesions

Overlooked or deliberately ignored adhesions create blind spots and can complicate or even prevent correct and fast instrument handling in the case of bleeding, which may appear more severe than it actually is owing to the endoscopic magnification. Adhesions should normally all be divided to allow a full view of the cavity.

If there are sail-like adhesions which make the initial optically controlled insertion of trocars impossible, the cavity can be probed with a fine needle on a syringe containing saline. Alternatively, fluoroscopy can be performed with the image intensifier, a technique used routinely by some pneumologists [26, 27], and this should reveal whether the selected site of entry is intrapleural or whether it would injure lung parenchyma.

Problems with the Endoscopic View

Misting of the Telescope. This problem can be prevented by prewarming the telescope or wiping it with anti-misting agent.

If the telescope becomes misted over in situ, it can be cleaned by retracting it into the trocar sleeve and rinsing it with the lateral taps or with the jet from the irrigation tube.

If the image nevertheless remains unclear, there may be condensed water between the camera and telescope connector.

Even small amounts of blood absorb a lot of light and significantly reduce the quality of the view in the thoracic cavity. We have found that it is best not to change the optical settings and position as far as possible to avoid focusing problems on top of the loss of light (set the camera focus before beginning the operation!). The blood can be diluted by alternate instillation and aspiration of irrigation solution.

Blood Seeping from the Entry Site. Blood which seeps from the entry site tends to run along the trocar sleeve to the inner opening. When the telescope is inserted, blood can then obstruct vision. This can be combatted by the following measures:

1. Always penetrating the thorax wall bluntly,
2. Applying anti-misting agent to the telescope, and
3. Rinsing the trocar sleeve when necessary with Ringer's solution, or
4. Cleaning the trocar sleeve with a gauze swab, much like cleaning a gun barrel.

Up to now, no ideal solution has been found for this problem.

Punctate Bleeding. Even punctate bleeding from the parietal pleura after dividing fresh, large-surface adhesions can reduce the lighting conditions for the telescope. This problem is best solved by regular irrigation and suction.

Thoracic Drainage

Thoracic drains should not be placed in lung fissures. Lung parenchyma can be sucked in and block the openings, stopping the action of the drain. When placing a drain intraoperatively, the displacement of the drain by the expanding lung must be taken into consideration, to make sure that the tip of the drain is at the required position on completion of the intervention.

Diameter of the Drain. Blood remnants and exudate soon block thin drains which should only be used as air drains when the pleural space is free of blood and exudate (uncomplicated pneumothorax after ligature, thoracoscopy for purely diagnostic inspection etc.). Even after a circumscribed biopsy, drainage tubes with a diameter of less than 24 Fr. should not be used.

Suction in the Thoracic Drainage System. The strength of the suction must be at least sufficient to exceed the negative pressure during inspiration. If pleural secretion moves toward the patient during inspiration, this is not the case. Intermittent formation of bubbles in the water seal is also an indication that the suction is inadequate or that there is a large pulmonary leak. If, despite continuous suction in the water seal and the absence of bubbles, a water level in the tubing system of the drainage bottle rises and falls, this points to a dead space or trapped lung.

Checking the Functions of the Thorax Drain on Completion of the Intervention. The sterile conditions at the operating table should be preserved until the correct functioning of the drainage system has been checked. If it is correctly installed, no more air should escape into the drainage bottle. If this is not the case, a further endoscopic examination of the lung should be considered so that any larger leaks that have been overlooked can be sealed.

The drains should never be clamped. Provided that the drainage bottle remains consistently below the height of the thorax, there is no risk for the patient.

Pain Caused by the Drain. The longer they are left, the more the drains cause unpleasant localized pain, which can best be alleviated by an additional adhesive tape to hold the drain in position. The patient should be asked to say which position is the most comfortable.

Removing the Thoracic Drain. It is best to remove the drain in the inspiratory position to prevent a sudden reflex inspiration by the patient.

Bedside Thoracoscopy

With the light source and the thoracoscope and without any other electrical equipment a simple, direct viewing thoracoscopy can be performed at the patient's bedside for diagnosis, aspiration of fluids or to perform pleurodesis. This bedside thoracoscopy is, for example, suitable for artificially ventilated patients in intensive care or prior to placing a thoracic drain through the incision.

19 The Current Situation and Prospects for the Future

The aim of minimally invasive surgery is to maintain the physical integrity of the patient as far as possible by reducing operative trauma. The resulting expectations such as the reduction in the time required for medical care and the patient's earlier reintegration in everyday life should be considered under two aspects: firstly as an undoubted benefit for the patient, but also as a way of encouraging the patient to play a more responsible role in his or her own therapy. Promoting the patient's insight into his or her own illness on the one hand, and minimizing the operative invasiveness on the other are the therapeutic aims which should determine the further development of this method.

In the light of this, the question posed recently during the opening speech at a congress by an exponent and pioneer of minimally invasive surgery gives grounds for serious thought: "Why should an arthroscopist, for example, continue to be instructed in general medicine or psychiatry, instead of being trained early on specifically for endoscopic tasks?" If this attitude is adopted, there is a danger that a surgical method that is still in its infancy but rich in promise will be doomed to come to a simplistic, technical dead end. The endoscopic surgeon is not some sort of cameraman, skilled electronics expert or talented fine mechanic. His primary role remains that of a physician active in the field of surgery. Recognition of a disease, selection of suitable therapy and above all sympathetic care of the patient require medical and not technical know-how. This means that a comprehensive medical training will certainly continue in the future to provide the basis for a surgeon's work. It is particularly important to maintain the standards of genuine and thorough medical knowledge and activity in a period in which new surgical avenues are being explored, since they must be carefully evaluated and compared with established, proven and successful surgical techniques.

Results can be quoted which illustrate the state of the art. If we compare the results of thoracoscopic therapy of spontaneous pneumothorax in our series with the treatment methods used previously in our hospital, endoscopic therapy performed according to consistent guidelines (although admittedly there are no long-term results) achieved significantly better results. The patients with idiopathic pneumothorax treated conservatively between 1980 and 1989 remained hospitalized for an average of 8 days per episode, and those with secondary pneumothorax an average of 24 days. The hospitalization of all patients treated thoracoscopically, regardless of aetiology, was 3.3 days. The recurrence rate in the conservatively treated group was 33%, and the current value in the thoracoscopic group is 4.8%.

Apart from the results and statistics related to morbidity and mortality, the early termination rates and number of conversions to thoracotomy also provide information about problems specific to the method. In our series, thoracoscopy was terminated eight times because of obliteration, and an unplanned conversion to thoracotomy was necessary nine times. In 14 cases, a second, unplanned intervention followed thoracoscopy (seven times involving a second thoracoscopy, twice a mini-thoracotomy, and five times a standard thoracotomy). The causes are listed in Table 17.

In terms of indications, the current possibilities and restrictions are reflected in Table 18. From a technical point of view, intrathoracic dissection will probably not remain the main problem, but rather the practical extraction of resected specimens suitable for precise pathological examination. Simply extending the incision defeats the object just as much as morcellating the specimen so that it can no longer be reconstructed. Accepted oncological guidelines must be adhered to. In

Table 17. Reasons for terminating thoracoscopy, intraoperative conversion or a second intervention after thoracoscopy

Cause	Termination	Conversion	Second intervention
Venous bleeding	−	+	−
Arterial bleeding	−	−	+
Obliteration	+	+	−
Infected fistula	−	+	+
Empyema	−	+	+
Trapped lung	−	+	+
Inconclusive biopsy	−	+	−
Overlooked pathology (e.g. atelectasis in organized haematoma)	−	−	+
Technically not possible (e.g. mediastinal biopsy)	−	+	−
Recurrence (e.g. malignant effusion, pneumothorax)	−	−	+

Table 18. Surgical thoracoscopy: current possibilities and limitations

Interventions	Clinical routine	Currently borderline	Experimental	Problems
Spontaneous pneumothorax	++			Long-term results, numbers of patients
Chylothorax	++			Numbers of patients
Pericardial surgery	+	+		Numbers of patients, long-term results
Extrapulmonary tumours	++	+		Extraction of resected material
Haematoma evacuation	++			Time thoracoscopy performed
Pleural empyema	++	++		Decortication on collapsed lung
Bronchopleural fistula	+	++		Time thoracoscopy performed
Peripheral carcinoma:				
Wedge resection	++	+	+	Oncological axioms
Segment resection		+	++	Thoracoscopic technique
Metastasis surgery		+	++	Thoracoscopic technique
Lobectomy			++	Thoracoscopic technique, instrument set
Pneumonectomy			++	Thoracoscopic technique, instrument set
Mediastinal lung cancer staging		(+)	++	Thoracoscopic technique

animal experiments, we successfully performed endoscopic lobectomy in five mini-pigs. Using the type of 12 mm trocar sleeve required for the Endo-GIA, we were able to remove the specimen easily and then reconstruct it after previously parcelling it into three pieces with the stapler.

With endoscopic surgery, we are witnessing the start of a new era. No matter how carefully and objectively we evaluate the usefulness and effectiveness of the method, and accepting that it is currently the subject of an often uncritical euphoria, there is nevertheless no going back. Our attitude must be such that we develop and promote inventiveness and imagination while keeping both feet firmly on the ground. As physicians it is our duty to investigate and test new methods for the benefit of our patients. It is increasingly our task to explain to the patient the wide variety of available methods and to choose the best possible therapy in the given situation.

References

1. Abbey Smith R (1957) The results of raising the resectability rate in operation for lung carcinoma. Thorax 12:79–86
2. Adler RH, Levinsky L (1978) Persistent chylothorax. J Thorac Cardiovasc Surg 76:859–864
3. Akaogi E, Kiyohumi M, Sohara Y, Endo S, Ishikawa S, Hori M (1989) Treatment of postoperative chylothorax with intrapleural fibrin glue. Ann Thorac Surg 48:116–118
4. American Thoracic Society (1962) Management of nontuberculous empyema. Am Rev Respir Dis 85:935–936
5. Austin EH, Flye MW (1979) The treatment of recurrent malignant pleural effusion. Ann Thorac Surg 28:190–203
6. Basmajian JV (1980) Grant's method of anatomy, 10th edn. Williams and Wilkins, Baltimore
7. Baumgartner WA, Mark JBD (1980) The use of thoracoscopy in the diagnosis of pleural disease. Arch Surg 115:420–421
8. Becker HP, Weidringer lW, Willy C, Hartel W, Blumel G (1991) Licht- und rasterelektronenmikroskopische Untersuchungen der Pleura. Langenbecks Arch Chir 376:295–301
9. Ben Isaac FE, Dimmons DH (1975) Flexible fiberoptic pleuroscopy in pleural and lung biopsy. Chest 67:573–576
10. Benninghof A (1985) Kreislauf und Eingeweide. In: Fleischhauer K (ed) Makroskopische und mikroskopische Anatomie der Menschen, vol 2, 13th/14th edn. Urban and Schwarzenberg, Munich
11. Bergqvist S, Nordenstam H (1966) Thoracoscopy and pleural biopsy in the diagnosis of pleurisy. Scand J Respir Dis 47:64–74
12. Bessone LN, Ferguson TB, Burford TH (1971) Chlyothorax. Ann Thorac Surg 12:527–550
13. Bethune N (1935) Pleural poudrage. A new technique for the deliberate production of pleural adhesions as a preliminary to lobectomy. J Thorac Cardiovasc Surg 4:251–261
14. Bloomberg AE (1978) Thoracoscopy in perspective. Surg Gynecol Obstet 147:433–443
15. Bogusch LK, Travin AA, Semenkow JL (1971) Transperikardiale Operationen an den Hauptbronchien und Lungengefäßen. Hippokrates, Stuttgart
16. Boniface E, Guerin JC (1989) Intérêt du talcage par thoracoscopie dans les traitements symptomatiques des pleurésies recidivantes. A propos de 302 cas. Rev Mal Respir 6:133–139
17. Boutin C (1991) Personal communication. Marseille

18. Boutin C, Astoul P, Seitz B (1990) The role of thoraco-
    scopy in the evaluation and management of pleural
    effusions. Lung 168 [Suppl]:1113–1121
19. Boutin C, Farisse P, Rex F, Viallat IR, Cargnino P
    (1989) La thoracoscopie doit-elle être un examen de
    routine en pratique pneumologique courante? Med Hyg
    42:2992–3000
20. Boutin C, Rey F, Viallat lR (1985) Etude randomisée de
    l'efficacité du talcage thoracoscopique et le l'instillation
    de tetracycline dans le traitement des pleurésies can-
    cereuses revidivantes. Rev Mal Respir 2:374
21. Boutin C, Viallat JR, Aelony Y (1991) Practical
    Thoracoscopy. Springer, Berlin Heidelberg New York
22. Boutin C, Viallat JR, Cargnino P, Farisse P (1981)
    Thoracoscopy in malignant pleural effusions. Am Rev
    Respir Dis 124:588–592
23. Brandt HJ (1964) Die Thorakoskopie bei Erkrankungen
    der Pleura und des Mediastinums. Internist 10:391–395
24. Brandt HJ (1981) Biopsie pulmonaire sous controle
    visuel. Poumon-Coeur 37:307–311
25. Brandt HJ, Kund H (1964) Die Leistungsfahigkeit
    der diagnostischen Thorakoskopie. Prax Pneumol 18:
    304–322
26. Brandt HJ, Loddenkemper R, Mai J (1983) Atlas der
    diagnostischen Thorakoskopie: Indikationen – Technik.
    Thieme, Stuttgart
27. Brandt HJ, Loddenkemper R, Mai J (1985) Atlas of
    diagnostic thoracoscopy. Thieme, Stuttgart
28. Branscheid D, Trainer S, Bulzebruck H, Vogt-Moykopf
    I (1988) Ergebnisse chirurgischer Therapie beim Spon-
    tanpneumothoraxn Langenbecks Arch Chir 2 [Suppl]:
    505–509
29. Brown EM, Kunjappan VE, Alexander GD (1984)
    Fentanyl/Alfentanyl for pelvic laparoscopy. Can Anaesth
    Soc J 31:251–154
30. Callahan JA, Seward JB, Tajik AJ, Holmes Dr, Smith
    HC, Reeder GS, Miller FA (1983) Pericardiocentesis
    assisted by twodimensional echocardiography. J Thorac
    Cardiovasc Surg 85:877–879
31. Canto A (1990) Macroscopic characteristics of pleural
    metastases arising from the breast and observed by diag-
    nostic thoracoscopy. Am Rev Respir Dis 142:616–618
32. Canto A (1981) Thoracoscopie: résultats dans les can-
    cers de la plèvre. Poumon-Coeur 37:235–239
33. Canto A, Blasco E, Casillas M, Zarza AG, Padilla J,
    Pastor J, Tarazona V, Paris F (1977) Thoracoscopy in
    the diagnosis of pleural effusion. Thorax 32:550–554
34. Canto A, Rivas J, Saumench J, Morera R, Moya J (1983)
    Points to consider when choosing a biopsy method in
    cases of pleurisy of unknown origin. Chest 84:176–179
35. Chernow B, Sahn SA (1977) Carcinomatous involve-
    ment of the pleura. Am J Med 63:695–702
36. Chowdhuri IK (1979) Percutaneous use of fiberoptic
    bronchoscope to investigate bronchopleurocutaneous
    fistula. Chest 75:203–204
37. Cova F (1928) Atlas thoracoscopicon. Sperling and
    Kupfer, Milan

38. DeCamp PT, Moseley PW, Scott ML, Hatch HB (1973) Diagnostic thoracoscopy. Ann Thorac Surg 16:79–84

39. Deslauriers J, Beaulieu M, Dufour C, Michaud P, Desprès JP, Lemieux M (1976) Mediastinopleuroscopy: a new approach to the diagnosis of intrathoracic diseases. Ann Thorac Surg 22:265–269

40. Deslauriers J, Beaulieu M, Desprès JP, Lemieux M Leblanc J, Desmeules M (1980) Transaxillary pleurectomy for treatment of spontaneous pneumothorax. Ann Thorac Surg 30:569–574

41. Dijkman JH, van der Meer JWM, Bakker W, Wever AMJ, van der Broek PJ (1982) Transpleural lung biopsy by the thoracoscopic route in patients with diffuse interstitial pulmonary disease. Chest 82:76–83

42. Dimitri WR (1987) Massive idiopathic spontaneous haemothorax – case report and literature review. Eur J Cardiothorac Surg 1:55–58

43. Driscoll PJ, Aronstam EM (1961) Experiences in the management of recurrent spontaneous pneumothorax. J Thorac Cardiovac Surg 42:174–178

44. Dubois F, Berthelot H, Levard H (1989) Cholecystectomie par coelioscopie. Presse Med 18:980–892

45. Elert O, Eigel P (1986) Treatment of idiopathic spontaneous pneumothorax: transthoracic endoscopic use of fibrin glue. In: Schlag G, Redl H (eds) Thoracic surgery cardiovascular surgery – fibrin sealant in operative medicine, vol 5. Springer, Berlin Heidelberg New York, pp 107–114

46. Enggist U (1979) Transpleurale Neurotomie. Rentsch AG, Trimbach-Olten

47. Errett LE, Wilson J, Chiu RC, Munro DD (1985) Wedge resection as an alternative procedure for peripheral bronchogenic carcinoma in poor risk patients. J Thorac Cardiovasc Surg 90:656–661

48. Faurschou P, Madsen F, Viskum K (1983) Thoracoscopy: influence of the procedure on some respiratory and cardiac values. Thorax 38:341–343

49. Faurschou P (1984) Induction of pneumothorax by means of the Veress canula. Eur J Respir Dis 65:547–549

50. Faurschou P (1985) Diagnostic thoracoscopy in pleuropulmonary infiltrates without pleural effusion. Endoscopy 17:21–25

51. Ferguson MK, Little AG, Skinner DB (1985) Current concepts in the management of postoperative chylothorax. Ann Thorac Surg 40:542–545

52. Fraser RS, Viloria JB, Wang NS (1980) Cardiac tamponade as a presentation of extracardiac malignancy. Cancer 45:1697–1704

53. Frey JG, Tschopp JM (1987) Chylothorax: traitement par pleurodèse au talc. Schweiz Med Wochenschr 117: 1624–1627

54. Furrer M. Inderbitzi R (1992) Pleurodeseverfahren beim malignen Pleuraerguss. Schweiz Med Wochenschr. 122: 181–188

55. Furrer M. Inderbitzi R (1992) Fallbericht: Endoskopische Resketion eines 5 cm grossen intrathorakalen Lipoms. Pneumologie 46

56. Gaensler EA (1956) Parietal pleurectomy for recurrent spontaneous pneumothorax. Surg Gynecol Obstet 102: 293–308

57. Getz SB. Beasley WE (1983) Spontaneous pneumothorax. Am J Surg 145:823–828

58. Glinz W (1981) Chest trauma – diagnosis and management. Springer, Berlin Heidelberg New York

59. Glover W. Chavis TV, Daniel TH, Kron IL, Spotnitz WD (1987) Fibrin glue application through the flexible fiber optic bronchoscope: closure of bronchopleural fistulas. J Thorac Cardiovasc Surg 93:470–472

60. Gobbel WG, Rhea WG, Nelson IA, Daniel RA (1963) Spontaneous pneumothorax. J Thorac Cardiovasc Surg 46:331–345

61. Good IT, Taryle DA, Maulitz RM, Kaplan RL, Sahn SA (1980) The diagnostic value of pleural fluid pH. Chest 78:55–59

62. Greschuchna D (1989) Thorakoskopie bei Brustwandprozessen. Pneumologie 2:119–121

63. Guerin JC, Boniface E (1990) Les méthodes de pleurodèse. Rev Prat 40:1854–1856

64. Guerin JC, Champel F, Biron E, Kalb IC (1985) Talcage pleural par thoracoscopie dans le traitement du pneumothorax. Etude d'une série de 109 cas traités en 3 ans. Rev Mal Respir 2:25–29

65. Guerin JC, Demolombe S, Brudon JR (1990) Sympatholyse thoracique par thoracoscopie. A propos de 15 cas. Rev Mal Respir 7:327–330

66. Guerin JV, Demolombe S, Brudon JR (1990) Sympatholyse thoracique par thoracoscopie. A propos de 15 cas. Ann Chir 44:236–238

67. Guerin JC. Martinat Y, Champel F, Berger C (1985) Obliteration d'une fistule bronchopleurale par laser YAG sous thoracoscope. Press Med 14:1245–1246

68. Gunnels JJ (1978) Perplexing pleural effusion. Chest 74:390–393

69. Guyton AC (1981) Textbook of medical physiology, 6th edn. Saunders, Philadelphia

70. Gwin E, Pierce G, Boggan M. Kerby G, Ruth W (1975) Pleuroscopy and pleural biopsy with the flexible fiber optic bronchoscope. Chest 67:527–531

71. Hafferl A (1969) Lehrbuch der topographischen Anatomie, 3rd edn. Springer, Berlin Heidelberg New York

72. Hankins JR, Miller EJ, McLaughlin JS (1978) The use of chest wall muscle flaps to close bronchopleural fistulas: experience with 21 patients. Ann Thorac Surg 25:491–499

73. Hansen MK, Kruse-Anderson S, Watt-Boolsen S, Andersen K (1989) Spontaneous pneumothorax and fibrin glue sealant during thoracoscopy. Eur J Cardiothorac Surg 3:512–514

74. Hartl H (1970) Mögliche und vermeidbare Fehler beim kindlichen Pleuraempyem. Arch Klin Chir 327:596

75. Hausheer FH, Yabro JW (1985) Diagnosis and treatment of malignant pleural effusion. Sem Oncol 12:54–75

76. Heindl W, Pridun N (1986) Endoscopic fibrin pleurodesis in complicated pneumothorax. In: Schlag G, Redl H (eds) Thoracic surgery – cardiovascular surgery – fibrin sealant in operative medicine, vol 5. Springer, Berlin Heidelberg New York, pp 89–94

77. Heine F (1957) Die Probeexzision aus Veränderungen im Thoraxraum und Lunge unter thorakoskopischer Sicht. Beitr Klin Tuberk 116:615–627

78. Houston MC (1987) Pleural fluid pH: diagnostic, therapeutic, and prognostic value. Am J Surg 154:333–337

79. Hovorka J, Kortila K, Erkola O (1989) Nitrous oxide does not increase nausea and vomiting following gynecological laparoscopy. Can J Anaesth 36:145–148

80. Hutter JA, Harari D, Braimbridge MV (1985) The management of empyema thoracis by thoracoscopy and irrigation. Ann Thorac Surg 39:517–520

81. Inderbitzi R, Althaus U (1991) Therapeutic thoracoscopy, a new surgical technique. Thorac Cardiovasc Surg 39 [Suppl]:35

82. Inderbitzi R, Furrer M, Althaus U (1991) Die thorakoskopische Behandlung des Spontanpneumothorax durch chirurgischen Leckverschluß. Schweiz Med Wochenschr 121 [Suppl]:18

83. Inderbitzi R, Furrer M. Klaiber Ch, Ris HB, Striffeler H, Althaus U (1992) Thoracoscopic wedge resection. Surg Endosc 6:189–192

84. Inderbitzi R, Furrer M, Striffeler H (1992) Die operative Thorakoskopie – Indikationen und Technik. Chirurg 63:334–341

85. Inderbitzi RGD, Furrer M, Striffeler H, Althaus U (1992) Thoracoscopic pleurectomy for treatment of complicated spontaneous pneumothorax. J Thorac Cardiovasc Surg (in press)

86. Inderbitzi R, Leupi F, Furrer M, Althaus U (1991) Die thorakoskopische Perikardfenestration – eine neue Methode zur Behandlung rezidivierender Perikardergüsse. Schweiz Med Wochenschr 121 [Suppl 36]:27

87. Inderbitzi R, Krebs T, Stirnemann P, Althaus U (1992) Treatment of postoperative chylothorax by fibrin glue under thoracoscopic view using local anesthesia. J Thorac Cardiovasc Surg 104:209–210

88. Inderbitzi R, Molnar J (1990) Erfahrungen in der diagnostischen und operativen Video-Endoskopie des Thoraxraumes. Schweiz Med Wochenschr 120:1965–1907

89. Jacobaeus HC (1912) Über Laparo- und Thorakoskopie. Beitr Klin Tuberk 25:185–354

90. Jacobaeus HC (1921) Die Thorakoskopie und ihre praktische Bedeutung. Dtsch Med Wochenschr 25:702–705

91. Jessen C, Sharma P (1985) Use of fibrin glue in thoracic surgery. Ann Thorac Surg 39:521–524

92. Jones JW, Kitahama A, Webb WR, McSwain N (1981) Emergency thoracoscopy. A logical approach to chest trauma management. J Trauma 21:280–284

93. Kaiser D (1987) Thoracoskopische Hämatomausräu-
    mung beim unvollstandig entleerten Hämatothorax.
    Hefte Unfallheikd 189:328–332
94. Kaiser D (1989) Fibrinklebung beim Spontanpneumo-
    thorax. Pneumologie 43:101–104
95. Kaiser D (1989) Indikation zur Thorakoskopie beim
    Pleuraempyem. Pneumologie 43:76–79
96. Kapsenberg PD (1981) Thoracoscopic biopsy under
    visual control. Poumon-Coeur 37:313–316
97. Klaiber Ch, Z'Graggen K, Metzger A, Leepin H (1990)
    Die laparoskopische Cholezystektomie. Unsere Erfah-
    rung in 20 Fällen. Schweiz Rundschau Med 79:787–790
98. Kralstein J, Frishman W (1987) Malignant pericardial
    diseases: diagnosis and treatment. Am Heart J 113:785–
    790
99. Lampson RS (1948) Traumatic chylothorax. A review of
    the literature and report of a case treated by mediastinal
    ligation of the thoracic duct. J Thorac Surg 17:778–791
100. Leff A, Hopewell PC, Costello J (1978) Pleural effusion
     from malignancy. Ann Intern Med 88:532–537
101. Lewis RJ, Kundermann PJ, Sisler GE, Mackenzie JW
     (1976) Direct diagnostic thoracoscopy. Ann Thorac Surg
     21:536–539
102. Lichter I (1974) Long-term follow-up of planned treat-
     ment of spontaneous pneumothorax. Thorax 29:32–37
103. Light RW, Girard WM, Jenkinson SG, George RB
     (1980) Parapneumonic effusions. Am J Med 69:507–512
104. Light RW (1985) Management of pleural effusions. In:
     Chretien J, Bignon J, Hirsch A (eds) The pleura in
     health and disease. Dekker, New York, pp 789–809
105. Linn RB (1958) Survey of the methods of bronchial
     stump closure. J Thorac Cardiovasc Surg 36:50
106. Little AG, Kremser PW, Wade IL, Levett JM, De-
     Meester TR, Skinner DB (1984) Operation for diagnosis
     and treatment of pericardial effusions. Surgery 96:738–
     744
107. LoCicero J III, Hartz RS, Frederiksen JW, Michaelis
     LL(1985) New application of the laser in pulmonary
     surgery: hemostasis and sealing of air leaks. Ann Thorac
     Surg 40:546–550
108. Loddenkemper R (1983) Diagnostik des Pleuraergusses.
     Intern Welt 10:293–301
109. Maasilta P, Vehmas T, Kivisaari L, Tammilehto L, Matt-
     son K (1991) Correlations beteween findings at computed
     tomography (CT) and at thoracoscopy/thoracotomy/
     autopsy in pleural mesothelioma. Eur Respir J 4:952–954
110. Maassen W (1972) Direkte Thorakoskopie ohne vor-
     herige oder mögliche Pneumothoraxanlage. Endoscopy
     4:95–98
111. Maisch B, Drude L (1991) Pericardioscopy – a new diag-
     nostic tool in inflammatory diseases of the pericardium.
     Eur Heart J 12 [Suppl]:2–6
112. Matzel W (1963) Diagnostische Thorakoskopie bei in-
     trathorakalen Rundherden. Z Tuberk 120:1–13
113. Miech G, Sroebner J, Razafindrazaka, Witz JP (1967)
     Les risques de la ponction biopsie transpariétale. L'ino-
     culation néoplastique. Presse Med 75:2803–2806

114. Migueres J, Jover A, Krempf M (1975) Notes sur les incidents et accidents de la biopsie pleurale à l'aiguille: l'ensemencement néoplastique da la paroi. Poumon-Coeur 31 :347–349

115. Miller JI, Hatcher CR (1978) Thoracoscopy: a useful tool in the diagnosis of thoracic disease. Ann Thorac Surg 26:68–72

116. Milson JW, Kron IL, Rheuban KS, Rodgers BM (1985) Chylothorax: an assessment of current surgical management. J Thorac Cardiovasc Surg 89:221–227

117. Mistal OM (1935) Endoscopie et pleurolyse. Masson, Paris

118. Moore DWO (1991) Malignant pleural effusion. Semin Oncol 18:59–61

119. Moritz E, Eckersberger F (1985) Endoskopische Klebung postoperativer Bronchusfisteln. Chirurg 56:125–127

120. Mortenson RL, Kvale PA, Lewis J, Groux N (1987) Tetracycline pleurodesis in recurrent pneumothorax of benign etiology. Am Rev Respir Dis 135:A57

121. Mouret P (1990) La chirurgie coelioscopique. Evolution ou revolution? Chirurgie 116:829–832

122. Mourout J, Benchimol D, Bernard JL, Tran A, Padovani B, Rampal P, Bourgeon A, Richelme H (1991) Exerese d'un kyste bronchogenique par video-thoracoscopie. Presse Med 20:1768–1769

123. Nadjafi AS, Konietzko N, Cegla UH, Matthys H (1976) La biopsie chirurgicale pleuropulmonaire chez les malades à haut risque pulmonaire. Bronchopneumologie 26:219–224

124. Oakes DD, Sherck JP, Brodsky JB, Mark JB (1984) Therapeutic thoracoscopy. J Thorac Cardiovasc Surg 87:269–273

125. Oldenburg FA Jr, Newhouse MT (1979) Thoracoscopy. A safe, accurate diagnostic procedure using the rigid thoracoscope and local anesthesia. Chest 75:45–50

126. Orringer MB (1988) Thoracic empyema – back to basics. Chest 93:901–902

127. Padhi RK, Lynn RB (1960) The management of bronchopleural fistulas. J Thorac Cardiovasc Surg 39:385–393

128. Pairolero PC, Arnold PB (1987) Bronchopleural fistula: management with muscle transposition. International trends in general thoracic surgery, vol 2. Saunders, Philadelphia

129. Patterson GA, Todd TRJ, Delarue NC, Ilves R, Pearson FG, Cooper JD (1981) Supradiaphragmatic ligation of the thoracic duct in intractable chylous fistula. Ann Thorac Surg 32:44–49

130. Person FG (1968) An evaluation of mediastinoscopy in the management of presumably operable bronchial carcinoma. J Thorac Cardiovasc Surg 55:617–625

131. Pérrisat J, Collet D, Belliard R (1989) Gallstones: laparoscopic treatment – intracorporeal lithotripsy, followed by cholecystostomy or cholecystectomy. A personal technique. Endoscopy 21:373–374

132. Peterson JA (1984) Recognition of intrapulmonary pleural effusion. Radiology 74:34

133. Pier A, Thevissen P, Ablassmaier B (1991) Die Technik der laparoskopischen Cholecystektomie am St. Josef Krankenhaus Linnich – Erfahrungen und Ergebnisse bei 200 Eingriffen. Chirurg 62:323–331

134. Potts DE, Tarylc DA, Sahn SA (1978) The glucose-pH relationship in parapneumonic effusions. Arch Intern Med 138:1378–1380

135. Pridun N (1989) A new biological implant for closure of bronchopleural fistulas. In: Waclawiczek HW (ed) Progress in fibrin sealing. Springer, Berlin Heidelberg New York

136. Prinz F, Klinner W (1953) Pathologisch-anatomische Untersuchungen zu Lungendekortikation. Langenbecks Arch Dtsch Z Chir 277:245–257

137. Radigan LR, Glover JL (1977) Thoracoscopy. Surgery 82:425–428

138. Ratliff JL, Johnson N, Clever JA (1977) Pleuroscopy and cautery control of intrathoracic haemorrhage with a flexible fiberoptic bronchoscope. Chest 71:216–217

139. Reddick EJ, Olsen DO (1989) Laparoscopic laser cholecystectomy. A comparison with minilap cholecystectomy. Surg Endosc 3:131–133

140. Ridley PD, Braimbridge MV (1991) Thoracoscopic debridement and pleural irrigation in the management of empysema thoracis. Ann Thorac Surg 51:461–464

141. Riedel H, Semm K (1980) The post-laparaoscopic syndrome. Geburtshilfe Frauenheilkd 40:635–643

142. Rodgers BM, Moazam F, Talbert JL (1979) Thoracoscopy in children. Ann Surg 189:176–180

143. Root B, Levy MN, Pollack S (1978) Gas embolism death after laparoscopy delayed by "trapping" in portal circulation. Anesth Analg 57:323–325

144. Rosato FE, Wallach MW, Rosato GF (1974) The management of malignant effusions from the breast cancer. J Surg Oncol 6:441–449

145. Rosenfeldt FL, McGibney D, Braimbridge MN, Watson DA (1981) Comparison between irrigation and conventional treatment for empyema and pneumonectomy space infection. Thorax 36:272–277

146. Sahn SA (1981) Pleural manifestation of pulmonary disease. Hosp Pract 16:73–79, 83–85, 89

147. Sarin CL, Nohl-Oser HC (1969) Mediastinoscopy. Thorax 24:585–588

148. Sattler A (1937) Zur Behandlung des Spontanpneumothorax mit besonderer Berücksichtigung der Thorakoskopie. Beitr Klin Tuberk 89:395–408

149. Sattler A (1937) Zur Pathogenese und Therapie des idiopathischen Spontanpneumothorax. Wien Arch Inn Med 30:77–96

150. Sattler A (1961) Die pleurale Biopsie. Ergebnisse und Bedeutung für die Praxis. Ciba Symp 9:109–121

151. Sattler A (1981) La thoracoscopie: intérêt therapeutique dans les syndromes pleuropulmonaires d'urgence et intérêt diagnostique. Poumon-Coeur 37:265–267

152. Schlag G, Redl H (1986) Principles of fibrin sealing. In: Schlag G, Redl H (eds) Thoracic surgery-cardiovascular

surgery – fibrin sealant in operative medicine, vol 5. Springer, Berlin Heidelberg New York, pp 3–59
153. Selle JG. Snyder WH, Schreiber JT (1973) Chylothorax. Indications for surgery. Ann Surg 177:245–249
154. Semm K (1983) Endoscopic appendectomy. Endoscopy 15:59–64
155. Senno A, Moallem S, Quijano ER, Adeyemo A, Clauss RH (1974) Thoracoscopy with the fiberoptic broncho-scope. A simple method in diagnosing pleuropulmonary diseases. J Thorac Cardiovasc Surg 67:606–611
156. Sgro M, Gorla A, Tacchi G, Iseppi P (1991) La toraco-scopia nella stadiazione dei tumori del polmone. Chir Ital 43:90–94
157. Shields TW (1989) Carcinoma of the lung. In: Shields TW (ed) General thoracic surgery. Lea and Febiger, Philadelphia, pp 890–943
158. Spalteberg W, Spanner R (1961) Handatlas der Anatomie des Menschen, 16th edn. Schettema and Holkema, Amsterdam
159. Stenzl W, Rigler B, Tscheliessnigg HK, Beitzke A, Metgler H (1983) Treatment of postsurgical chylothorax with fibrin glue. Thorac Cardiovasc Surg 31:35–36
160. Striffeler H, Inderbitzi R, Furrer M (1992) Die diagnos-tische Videothorakoskopie. Schweiz Med Wochenschr 122 [Suppl 44]:7
161. Swierenga JM, Wagenaar JP, Bergstein P (1974) The value of thoracoscopy in the diagnosis and treatment of diseases affecting the pleura and lung. Pneumologie 151:11–18
162. Swierenga J (1978) Atlas of thoracoscopy. Boeringer, Ingelheim am Rhein
163. Toomes H, Linder A (1989) Thorakoskopische Sym-pathektomie bei Hyperhydrosis. Pneumologie 43:107–108
164. Torre M, Belloni P (1989) Nd – YAG laser pleurodesis through thoracoscopy: new curative therapy in spon-taneous pneumothorax. Ann Thorax Surg 47:887–889
165. Tschopp JM, Evéquoz D, Karrer W, Aymon E, Naef AP (1990) Successful closure of chronic bronchopleural fistula by thoracoscopy after failure of endoscopic fibrin glue application and thoracoplasty. Chest 97:745–746
166. Van Berkel M, Dijkman JH (1990) Tension subcuta-neous emphysema. A case report. Neth J Med 36:25–28
167. Vanderschueren RG (1981) Le talcage pleural dans le pneumothorax spontane. Poumon-Coeur. 37:273–276
168. Vanderschueren RGJRA (1990) The role of thoraco-scopy in the evaluation and management of pneumo-thorax. Lung 168 [Suppl]:1122–1125
169. Verhandlungsbericht – Thorakoskopie-Symposium (1989) Berlin, Lungenklinik Heckeshorn 1987. Pneumo-logie 2/43
170. Vietri F, Tosato F, Passaro U, Vasapollo L, Tombolini P, Lavalle G, Guglielmi R (1991) L'impiego della colla di fibrina umana nella patologia fistolosa del pulmone. G Chir 12:399–402

171. Virkkula L (1987) Bronchopleural fistula: omental pedicle for treatment. International trends in general thoracic surgery, vol 2. Saunders, Philadelphia

172. Viskum K, Enk GB (1981) Complications of thoracoscopy. Poumon-Coeur 37:25–28

173. Viskum K (1989) Contraindications and complications to thoracoscopy. Pneumology 43:55–57

174. Voellmy W (1981) Résultats diagnostiques de la thoracoscopie dans les affections du poumon et de la plèvre. Poumon-Coeur 37:67–73

175. Vogel B, Mall W (1990) Thorakoskopische Perikardfensterung – diagnostische und therapeutische Aspekte. Pneumologie 44:184–185

176. Vogt–Moykopf I, Krumhaar H, Lüllig M, Moshtagi M (1974) Zur Diagnostik und prognostischen Bedeutung des Pleuraergusses bei Malignitätsverdacht. Thoraxchirurgie 22:398–401

177. Wakabayashi A (1989) Thoracoscopic ablation of blebs in the treatment of recurrent or persistent spontaneous pneumothorax. Ann Thorac Surg 48:651–653

178. Waclawiczek HW, Chmeuzek F, Koller I (1987) Endoscopic sealing of infected bronchus stump fistulae with fibrin following lung resections: experimental and clinical experience. Surg Endosc 1:99–102

179. Wakabayashi A, Brenner M, Wilson AF, Tadir Y, Berns M (1990) Thoracoscopic treatment of spontaneous pneumothorax using carbon dioxide laser. Ann Thorac Surg 50:786–789

180. Weese JL, Schouten JT (1982) Pleural peritoneal shunts for the treatment of malignant pleural effusions. Surg Gynecol Obstet 154:391–392

181. Weissberg D, Kaufman M (1980) Diagnostic and therapeutic pleuroscopy. Experience with 127 patients. Chest 78:732–735

182. Weissberg D, Kaufmann M. Schwecher I (1981) Pleuroscopy in clinical evaluation and staging of lung cancer. Poumon-Coeur 37:241–243

183. Werdermann K, Greschuchna D, Maassen W (1974) Ergebnisse chirurgischer Lungen und Pleurabiopsien. Thor Chir 22:453–456

184. West JB (1977) Regional differences in the lung. Academic, New York

185. Wickham JEA (1987) The new surgery. Br Med J 295:1581

186. Wihelm IM (1990) La place de la pleuroscopie dans le bilan préoperatoire du cancer bronchique. Ann Chir 44:139–142

187. Withers JN, Fishback CM, Kiel PV, Hannon JL (1964) Spontaneous pneumothorax: suggested etiology and comparison of treatment methods. Am J Surg 108:772–776

188. Wittmoser R (1959) Thoracoscopic sympathectomy in circulatory disorders of the arm. Langenbecks Arch Chir 292:318–323

189. Wittmoser R (1961) Thoraxchirurgie: Fehler und Gefahren der thorakoskopischen Deneveration. Chir Prax 1:79–92

190. Wittmoser R (1978) Operative Methode zur Behandlung des krankhaften Schwitzens (Hyperhidrosis). Ärztl Kosmetol 6:2–12
191. Wittmoser R (1984) Treatment of sweating and blushing by endoscopic surgery. Clin Neurol Neurosurg 86:122–124
192. Wittmoser R (1984) Possibilities of using sympathectomy for treatment of pain syndromes. Appl Neurophysiol 47:203–207
193. Woodring JH (1984) Recognition of pleural effusion on supine radiographs: how much fluid is required? Am J Roentgenol 142:59–64

Index

D. Gossot, P. Kleinmann, J. F. Levi (Eds.)

Surgical Thoracoscopy

With contributions by numerous experts

Preface by D. J. Sugarbaker

1992. XIII, 111 pp. 121 figs. ISBN 3-540-59577-5

In the first part of the work the instrumentation and the basic techniques are described. The main procedures in pleural, lung, mediastinal and esophageal pathology are then detailed. Their indications and results are discussed.

The medical data of interest for those surgeons who might treat pleural diseases through thoracoscopy are given. In case of opposite or complementary techniques coexisting for a same topic, each technique is dealt with by an author experienced in it.

C. Boutin, J. R. Viallat, Y. Aelony

Practical Thoracoscopy

With the collaboration of F. Rey

Foreword by R. W. Light

1991. XI, 107 pp. 70 figs. (46 in color), 13 tabs. ISBN 3-540-52369-3

This practical book has two main goals. The first is to show that thoracoscopic techniques are simple, require only short-term hospitalization, use only basic equipment, and are within the capability of not only surgeons, but other specialists as well. The second is to emphasize the exciting aspects of this endoscopic procedure with its wide variety of findings in the pleura, the diaphragm, the lung, and the mediastinum.

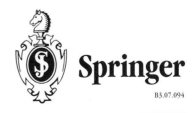

Springer

Springer-Verlag
and the Environment

We at Springer-Verlag firmly believe that an international science publisher has a special obligation to the environment, and our corporate policies consistently reflect this conviction.

We also expect our business partners – paper mills, printers, packaging manufacturers, etc. – to commit themselves to using environmentally friendly materials and production processes.

The paper in this book is made from low- or no-chlorine pulp and is acid free, in conformance with international standards for paper permanency.

Printing: Saladruck, Berlin
Binding: Buchbinderei Lüderitz & Bauer, Berlin